Diabulimia:
Diabetes + Eating Disorders
What It Is and How to Treat It

A Guide for Individuals and Families
A Tool for Health Personnel

W9-CFG-834

By
Grace Huifeng Shih, R.D. M.S.

Editors:
Bruce Buckingham, MD
Rosanna Fiallo-Scharer, MD

Library of Congress: LCCN 2011902733

Graphic Illustrator: Matthew Sheppard

First Edition
To learn more about the author: www.GraceNutrition.org

To Purchase: http://www.createspace.com/3562632

Or www.amazon.com

http://www.amazon.com/DIABULIMIA-Diabetes-Disorders-Individuals-Personnel/dp/1460930983/ref=sr_1_1?s=books&ie=UTF8&qid=1301640503&sr=1-1

Acknowledgments

First and foremost, I would like to thank Dr. Rosanna Fiallo-Scharer. She meticulously went through my manuscript page by page and word by word. Her dedication to the subject of diabetes combined with eating disorders is admirable. I deeply appreciate the devotion we share to the cause of helping those who suffer and educate those who treat this deadly dual condition. My gratitude is boundless to Dr. Bruce Buckingham, who is recognized worldwide for his breakthrough research. Even with his multiple research projects and patients by the hundreds, he found it in his heart and his schedule to support me in making sure this book is valuable and informative.

I am grateful to Betsy Kunselman, RN, CDE who sits right beside me at work, always nurturing me and sharing her knowledge, wisdom and expertise in treating type 1 diabetes mellitus. She is the most generous of colleagues, freely and selflessly giving with no expectation of anything in return. I am thankful for Dr. Darrel Wilson for his unending belief in me, and his support of me by providing resources. He has encouraged me, built my confidence in this project, wanting me to be the best I can be in the field of diabulimia. I thank Dr. Caroline Buckway who creates a relaxing and happy working environment. She allows me to make mistakes, from that I am able to grow and thrive in the field of diabetes. I am also delighted and grateful to work with Dr. Tandy Aye. It is such a pleasure and honor to be part of the diabetes team at Lucile Packard Children's Hospital (LPCH), Stanford Medical Center.

To Dr. Douglas Frederick, well known ophthalmologist, I express gratitude for coaching me in the area of diabetic retinopathy. I thank neurologist Dr. Susan Hwang who guided me as I wrote the section on diabetic neuropathy. To my beloved son-in-law, Dr. Steve Kim, nephrologist, I offer my gratitude for his encouragement and guidance in the area of diabetic nephropathy

And I thank Linda Johnson, Kelli Hall, Kristin Lund, Christina De La Rosa and Patricia Laurel for their hard work. Their contribution to this book is more valuable than they could imagine. I thank all the staff members of South Bay clinic, LPCH. Their genuine kindness to me creates a joyful work place for me.

Everything I know in the field of eating disorders I have learned from Dr. Iris Litt, Dr. Hans Steiner (two founders of the eating disorders program at LPCH), Dr. James Lock, Dr. Cynthia Kapphahn, Dr. Seth Ammerman, and Tom McPherson. I am extremely blessed to have them as my lifetime mentors and my dear friends. Particularly, Dr. James Lock has shepherded me and led me through the psychological complexity of diabulimia. He and Dr. Julie Collier coached me through the section of psychology in this book. I express my gratitude.

I thank Dr. Neville Golden and Phyllis Dejon, RN, who went through the treatment sections in this book checking for accuracy and workability in the hospital. More gratitude goes to Dr. Ann Goebel-Fabri, psychologist at Joslin clinic, who shared her studies and research; and to Theresa Garner who led me to the vital resources. To Dr. John Kerner, I express thanks for a steady support of many years in any professional subject.

I am humbled to serve on the board of the Eating Disorder Resource Center with a group of dynamic women: Janice Bremis, Denise Bridges, Kathleen Davidson, Dr. Seham El-Diwany, (whose inspiring devotion to patients with eating disorders and their families I try to emulate.), Candace Ford Gray (who teaches me the nuts and bolts of book publishing) and Nancy Shardell.

Last but not least, my gratitude goes to all the psychotherapists and their families who have been such a blessing to me, both professionally and personally. To me, they are family: Dr. Anthony Atwell, Dr. Andrea Ancha, Dr. Betsy Cregger, Dr. John Greene, Dr. Christina Halsey, Susan Hamlin, Ann Martini, Dr. Thomas Miller, Dr. Fawn Powers, Dr. Rebecca Powers (who leads me to my career of private practice), Dr. Veronica Saleh, Dr. Judith Segel, Carla Snyder, Dr. Melissa Sorci, Dr. Anne Takahashi, Dr. Gale Uhl and the late Dr. Larry Gibson. Dr. Tonja Krautter, who inspired me and started me on the path to book writing, has been kind to lend her support through every step of my writing process. I could not be more proud of an endorsement from her.

Special thanks to my daughter, Dr. Alice Chen Kim. She is my hero who shows me that: there is no unreachable star, and there is no impossible dream.

This book is dedicated:

To my incredible husband, John Sheehan, who adores me and spoils me regardless of which stage of women's hormonal tumult I may be going through. His overwhelming love enables me to live out my compassion for others, and my passion to help them.

To those who suffer from diabulimia: My concern for your well being is the driving force behind this book. Without your stories, your fear, your struggle, your desire to be well and your amazing courage, this book would not exist.

CONTENTS

Chapter 1

AN OUTCRY

Mary, age 28
"I have diabulimia. Why doesn't anyone take it seriously?"

"I am 28 years old with a dual condition called diabulimia. No one seems to be taking it seriously. When I was diagnosed with type 1 diabetes I was 16. That's the age when I should have been thinking about getting a car, driving to ball games, going to parties. Instead, I was in a hospital room and my Mom was crying her eyes out when they broke the news to us. My little brother took away the bag of cookies he brought from home giving me this "I'm sorry" look. I was numb, I didn't know what to think, or what to expect. Did it mean I couldn't go out for pizza or ice cream with my friends anymore? I got on insulin, and in just a few months, I had gained 15 pounds. And I was already 20 pounds overweight! I was so mad--not sad but mad. I decided to cut back on the insulin and not tell anyone.

Twelve years went by, and by then I was not only mad, but also sad and depressed. Oh, sure, I could go out with my friends and pig out. I could drink alcohol like there was no tomorrow, and I did for a couple of weeks when I turned 21. I could even stuff myself with as many cookies as I wanted. And as long as I didn't take my insulin I could still squeeze into my size 8 jeans.

Now I can hardly walk--some of my toes have turned purple and some are completely black. I was told I would lose my feet and maybe even my legs too. But I am only 28! I want to date, to get married and to have kids. Why didn't someone tell me this would happen? Why didn't anybody help me when I was 18, 20 or 22?"

NOBODY TOLD MARY THAT CUTTING BACK
ON INSULIN COULD EVENTUALLY RESULT IN
THE LOSS OF LIMBS.

Chapter 2

WHAT IS DIABULIMIA?

Diabulimia is an eating disorder in which people with type 1 diabetes deliberately give themselves less insulin than they need. They do this for the purpose of weight loss. When insulin is omitted, calories are purged through glucosuria, the loss of glucose through the urine. Individuals with diabulimia manipulate insulin ("a medication") as an inappropriate compensatory behavior to prevent weight gain. This is one of the criteria of bulimia nervosa per *DSM IV (Diagnostic and Statistical Manual of Mental Disorders-Fourth Edition)*.

Clinicians have yet to officially define the frequency and duration of insulin omission required for this dual condition to be diagnosed as a disorder. Some propose the following definition: Reducing or omitting insulin doses at least twice a week; a reduction of the prescribed insulin by over one quarter for more than three months for the purpose of weight loss.

The term "diabulimia" began to surface among public and health communities through news, magazines, and health journals in the summer of 2007. Yet individuals on websites, in blogs and in chat rooms had been using the word "diabulimia" for years before that.

The Clinician's Term: ED-DMT1

Most clinicians do not like the term diabulimia. In September of 2008, clinicians with an interest and expertise in eating disorders and diabetes held an international conference in Minneapolis, Minnesota. During that conference they recommended that the term ED-DMT1 be used to designate those with an eating disorder combined with type 1 diabetes mellitus. However, because the term diabulimia is more familiar to the public and to concerned individuals, and has been commonly used to refer to the condition, diabulimia will be used throughout this book.

Chapter 3

THE NECESSITY OF INSULIN
FOR TYPE 1 DIABETES

Type 1 diabetes is the result of autoimmune β cell destruction, leading to severe or absolute insulin deficiency. Insulin is a hormone produced by β cells of the pancreas which permits glucose from the bloodstream to go to the cells, muscles and liver by binding with the glucose transporter called GLUT 4.

Virtually all cells in the body use glucose as their main energy source. Without insulin, those GLUT 4 glucose transporters are not signaled to move to the cell surface, and glucose cannot enter the cells. This causes the cells to starve and eventually resort to alternative fuel sources through the breakdown of fat into "ketones" which can lead to diabetic ketoacidosis, a potentially fatal condition.

Insulin also plays an important role in glycogenesis, the process whereby glucose is stored as glycogen in the liver and muscles. Glycogen is the source of fuel during fasting and exercise.

How Does Lack of Insulin Cause Weight Loss?

Lack of insulin leads to decreased glucose uptake by the cells, resulting in increased blood glucose. When the concentration of glucose in the blood exceeds a threshold of between 160-180mg/dL, glucose is "dumped" into the urine. The classical symptoms of polyuria (frequent urination), polydipsia (increased thirst) and polyphagia (increased hunger) result.

When the blood glucose level is consistently above 250mg/dL, large quantities of glucose are lost into the urine instead of being utilized in the cells for energy; as a result weight loss can be significant since the loss of glucose is also the loss of calories.

Kathy, age 21:
"I wanted to wear a size 6 bridesmaid's gown, so I cut my insulin back."

> *"When my brother got married, they were having this huge wedding with six bridesmaids! The dresses were beautiful. I usually wear a size 10, but all the other dresses were being ordered in size 6's and 8's--one girl even ordered a size 2! I refused to be the one wearing the biggest bridesmaid's gown at my own brother's wedding. When my future sister in law asked what size to order for me, I said "size 6. " I knew the only way I could fit in that dress was to cut way back on my insulin and I had six weeks to do it. It is just amazing that I lost 19 pounds and the size 6 gown fit perfectly --- just by cutting back on insulin without even worrying much about what I ate. Of course, I kept doing it after the wedding -- I wanted to stay thin. I knew it was stupid but I didn't know just how dangerous it was."*

The Prevalence of Diabulimia: How Many Are Suffering?

Cases of type 1 diabetes mellitus combined with eating disorders have been published since early 1980's. In the past few years the prevalence of this dangerous combination has ranged from 11 percent to 39 percent among those with type 1 diabetes depending on the sample size, the age group, and the geographic area. Studies were conducted via self-report questionnaires and assessment tools such as *Assessing Health and Eating Disorders among Adolescents with Diabetes*; *Eating Disorder Inventory*; *Bulimic Investigatory Test* or the *Diabetes Eating Problem Survey*.

Since some people fail to return surveys and others are not completely truthful during their interviews, researchers believe that the actual number of individuals who have type 1 diabetes combined with an eating disorder could be much higher than the percentages indicated in the studies. Recent research data suggests that women with type 1 diabetes mellitus are 2.4 times more at risk for developing an eating disorder than are women without diabetes.

THE RATIO OF DIABULIMIA AMONG
WOMEN TO MEN IS 10:1.

Chapter 4

WHO IS AT RISK?
DIABULIMIA WARNING SIGNS

Warning Sign 1: Consistently High Hemoglobin A1c

Individuals who suffer from diabulimia often experience hyperglycemia, with an average glucose level of over 200mg/dL and HbA1c over 10.5% being common. The American Diabetes Association currently recommends maintaining HbA1c levels at or below 7.0% (eAG=154mg/dL).

(glycosylated hemoglobin) **or eAG** *(estimated average glucose).*
HbA1c (percent) x 28.7 – 46.7 = eAG (mg/dL)

Glycosylated hemoglobin or HbA1c tests provide an index to the average blood glucose level over a period of approximately three months. It is expressed as a percentage. Estimated average glucose uses the same units (mg/dL) that individuals see routinely when testing with their home glucose meter.

HbA1c x 28.7-46.7=eAG

Hemoglobin A1c (%)	eAG (mm/dL)	Hemoglobin A1c (%)	eAG (mm/dL)
6.0	126	11.5	283
6.5	140	12.0	298
7.0	154	12.5	312
7.5	169	13.0	326
8.0	183	13.5	341
8.5	197	14.0	355
9.0	212	14.5	369
9.5	226	15.0	384
10.0	240	15.5	398
10.5	255	16.0	412
11.0	269	16.5	427

High HbA1c may be also associated with other conditions:

Depression

According to studies, 25 percent of individuals with type 1 diabetes suffer from the co-morbidity of depression. The group of individuals experiencing depression may not be motivated to take care of themselves; hence their HbA1c may be high. These people may not necessarily have eating disorders.

Poor Diabetes Management

Some adolescents going through a transitional stage wish to be in charge of their own diabetes management, rather than be dependent on their parents. However, if their focus is on their peers and social gatherings, rather than checking blood glucose or injecting insulin, they may neglect their diabetes management and experience consistent hyperglycemia; yet, they may not have an eating disorder.

There are also other causes leading to high HbA1c, for example: the use of steroid medications such as prednisone due to chronic medical condition.

NOT EVERYBODY WITH A HIGH HBA1C HAS DIABULIMIA.

The key risk factors in diabulimia are distorted body image and irregular eating behavior.

When type 1 diabetes mellitus and eating disorders do co-exist, the two conditions become enmeshed and entrenched. The diabetes requires insulin dependence; the eating disorder "sees" insulin as the enemy. As body image distortion and irregular eating behavior increase, so does poor diabetes management.

Warning Sign 2: Body Image Concerns.

Individuals with diabulimia may be underweight, overweight, or within a good weight range. No matter their weight, they will show significantly increased body dissatisfaction and be driven to be thinner. A 2010 survey of normal weight teenagers indicated that more than 35 percent of girls and 14 percent of boys consider themselves to be overweight. Among individuals with type 1 diabetes, at least one third of the population is very concerned about body image and the need to lose weight. Desire for weight loss and fear of weight gain contribute to a high risk of calorie purging through insulin manipulation.

People may not be completely honest in divulging their true situation and disordered eating behavior. The health personnel must use skillful interview techniques to identify risks of eating disorders for early intervention. (See Chapter 5.)

Warning Sign 3: Irregular Eating Patterns

The eating behavior of individuals with diabulimia is very similar to the eating pattern found in those with bulimia nervosa.

- **Vicious eating cycles**

Individuals with diabulimia may restrict food intake, skip meals, and eliminate sweets and fats with the intention of losing weight. This behavior is followed by intense overeating which results in remorse and guilt. That triggers even more drastic eating deprivation, and/or the decision to avoid taking insulin. Then the vicious cycle repeats.

12

Some restrict food and insulin in order to lose weight, and many demonstrate weight loss for a period of time. However, the erratic eating behavior slows their metabolism, and lasting weight loss seldom occurs. When they also have diabetes and omit insulin, the glucosuria provides an additional method of caloric purging.

- **History of on-and-off dieting**

The risk for using insulin omission to lose weight is much higher if the individuals have tried various weight loss diets. A recent study (2010) of women aged 25-45 indicated that over 74.5 percent of those studied had been on a diet at least once in their lifetime; yet only 26 percent out of 4,000 women had a BMI, Body Mass Index over 25 (10 -15 lbs over median body weight). Half of the respondents on a random college student survey (3,8204 students) said they were trying to lose weight, even though only 28 percent were overweight. The most stunning study indicated that 40 percent of today's children as young as age nine have already tried dieting to some extent.

- **Discomfort in eating around other people**

Because of their irregular eating behavior, individuals with diabulimia prefer not to eat around other people, especially when they have the urge to overeat. Even if they join the family at the dinner table, they will choose foods with fewer calories and eat small portions.

Lisa, age 15:
"No one would believe what I eat when I'm alone."

> *"I don't want anybody to see me eating. If I have to eat with my family, I just eat bits of this or that and say I'm not hungry. I plan things so I hardly ever have to eat breakfast or dinner when anybody is around. I don't even like to eat with my friends at school. At home after school, when no one is around, I eat non stop. I can polish off a whole package of cookies or a big bag of chips. It gets worse when I'm bored."*

- **Hoarding food**

Without insulin, nutrients cannot get to the cells. When the cells need nutrition, the individual feels hungry. To satisfy that hunger, the person craves food. But those with diabulimia may feel guilty, defeated, or ashamed if they lose control over their eating in front of other people. Therefore, they may hoard foods and eat alone during weak moments.

Helen's Mom:
"Why does my daughter hide food in her room?"

> *"My daughter is always complaining that she is too fat. But she isn't really. Losing more weight is the most important thing in life to her, like an obsession. So when I started finding candy wrappers under her bed, and crumbs, I couldn't understand it. I would notice things were missing out of the cabinets, or the refrigerator. First I couldn't understand why Helen would hide what she was eating. And then I couldn't understand how she stayed so thin. Later we found out she hadn't been taking all her insulin."*

- **Reading ingredients or counting calories and fat grams**

Some disordered eaters become obsessed with counting calories, and refuse to eat foods containing high fat content. Some simply won't eat anything unless they know its exact calorie count. That's why those with eating disorders may stay away from foods like lasagna, casseroles, and certain meals Mom cooks or a restaurant serves. They may insist on knowing exactly what the ingredients are in what they're eating, so they can calculate the precise calorie count.

Nancy's friend:
"I hate going to a restaurant with her."

> *I have known Nancy since we were in elementary school when she was diagnosed with diabetes. I used to go with her to the nurse's office to take her insulin shots and we became best friends. These days, Nancy has to know the exact calorie count of everything she eats. If she has an apple she will try to figure out its diameter, so she can count every single calorie. It can be embarrassing to go to a restaurant with her because she has to interrogate the waiter and ask questions about everything and what's in it, and how it is cooked. When she comes over for dinner, she'll ask "how much oil did you put in it?" I wonder if Nancy has an eating disorder. "*

- **Fluctuating weight or acute weight loss**

Wild swings of weight fluctuation or evidence of acute weight loss may be indicative of some form of irregular eating.

Warning Sign 4: Exercising Compulsively

Appropriate regular exercise is a healthy practice, but compulsive exercise is another way some people "purge" calories. Some of them exercise after eating as another compensatory behavior to prevent weight gain. Some are anxious without the rigid daily exercise ritual, and some feel guilty if they don't exercise.

Warning Sign 5: Irregular or nonexistent menses, amenorrhea

High HbA1c levels have been reported to cause irregular menses, cessation of menstrual periods, and delayed puberty due to interference with the function of the brain (hypothalamic-pituitary-gonadal axis). In addition, inadequate glycemic control also results in **slow growth velocity and delayed development in some adolescents.**

Warning Sign 6: Repeat episodes of DKA, diabetic ketoacidosis

Warning Sign 7: Unwillingness to follow through with appointments

Due to the unwillingness of the individuals to get well (thinking it will mean weight gain) and the lack of awareness and information for the families, follow-up treatment for diabulimia is a great challenge.

Warning Sign 8: Doubtful blood glucose monitoring

If the numbers shown in blood glucose meters seem too good to be true, they are. Manipulation of blood glucose results should be suspected when the average blood glucose on the meter and the HbA1c are largely mismatched.

Chapter 5

DIFFERENT RESPONSES FOR DIABULIMIA, DEPRESSION, OR UNCONTROLLED BLOOD GLUCOSE

Questions to Identify Body Image Dissatisfaction

Question	Possible Answer	Explanation
1. "How much do you weigh?"	**Most would answer:** *"I am not sure"* or *"I just got weighed by your staff"*.	This question is to reveal the individual's perception of his/her weight, even though the clinicians already have the numbers.
	People with eating disorders might answer: *"133.5 lbs or 60.8kg"*, *"Are you sure your scale is right? It's a half pound more than my scale showed this morning"*.	Answers like this are a good indication of being overly concerned about body weight.

2. "How much do you think you should weigh?"	Normal answer for person who is 15 pounds overweight: *"I would like to get down to_____. (realistic, healthy weight)*	The answer to this question gives care taker a clear understanding of one's body image.
	Individual with depression: *"I don't know and I don't care."*	
	Individuals with eating disorders are likely to state that they need to weigh far less than their current weight and even far less than a healthy weight for them.	
3. "How often do you weigh yourself?"	**Most would answer:** *"Whenever I'm at my doctor's office"*, or *"every so often when I see a scale"*.	
	Individuals with eating disorders weigh daily and some even weigh themselves several times a day.	
4. "Do you see yourself as underweight, overweight, or just right?"	*"I feel fat and I look fat. I wish people would stop telling me I'm too skinny!"* *From someone with eating disorders.*	Health Personnel may ask this question for someone who is underweight.

Questions to Identify Irregular Eating Patterns

Question	Possible Answer	Explanation
1. "How many meals and snacks do you eat a day?"		The answers to these questions can identify someone who is uncomfortable eating with others, and someone who is restricting foods. People with depression may also not join the family at meals, but will eat all foods with small amounts.
2. "Have you been on a diet? Are you on a diet now?"		
3. "Do you follow a meal plan?"		
4. "Do you eat with your family at dinner? Do you eat with your friends at lunch?"		

5. "What kind of milk do you drink? Whole milk, 2 percent, or non-fat?"	Individual with depression or uncontrolled blood glucose: *"I don't know. I think it's a red container"*, or *"Whatever we have at home"*. Individual with an eating disorder would avoid drinks or foods with fat.	Questions 5 and 6 could further identify how drastically they are restricting fats or counting calories
6. "How many calories are in an apple?"	Individuals with an eating disorder know the exact number of calories for a medium size apple and many other foods. Individuals with depression will eat anything without knowing the calories, but only have a very small amount. Individuals with uncontrolled diabetes don't even think about how many calories foods have.	

A Checklist for Diabulimia Risk Factors

Question	Answers	At Risk for Diabulimia	
"How much do you weigh?"		YES	NO
"How much do you think you should weigh?"		YES	NO
"How often do you weigh yourself?"		YES	NO
"Do you see yourself as overweight?"		YES	NO
"Have you ever been overweight?"		YES	NO
"What is the best way to lose weight?"		YES	NO
"How does insulin affect your weight?"		YES	NO
"How often do you take less insulin than your food and blood sugar require?"		YES	NO

"When was your last menstrual period?"		YES	NO
"How often are your menstrual periods?"		YES	NO
"Have you ever been on a diet?"		YES	NO
"Are you on a diet now?"		YES	NO
"Do you follow a meal plan?"		YES	NO
"Do you eat with your family and friends?"		YES	NO
"Do you skip meals?"		YES	NO
"Do you count calories?" or "How many calories are in an apple?"		YES	NO
"Do you count fat grams?" or "What kind of milk do you drink?"		YES	NO
"Have you ever taken diet pills or laxatives?"		YES	NO

"Have you ever felt like you binged?"		YES	NO
"Have you ever felt the urge to make yourself throw up after eating?"		YES	NO
"How much do you exercise a day or a week?"		YES	NO
"Do you feel guilty if you don't exercise?"		YES	NO

Chapter 6

THE CONSEQUENCES OF DIABULIMIA
AND THE PEOPLE WHO SUFFER

Consequence I: Diabetic Ketoacidosis and Death

When insulin administration is restricted, the cells cannot obtain glucose for energy. The liver then produces glucose through the process of glycogenolysis (breakdown of glycogen to glucose) and gluconeogenesis (the formation of glucose from non-carbohydrate sources such as amino acids or fatty acids).

In the absence of insulin, muscle cells obtain most of their energy supply from ketones via ketogenesis (breakdown of fatty acids to ketones). As ketones are being produced, hydrogen ion concentration increases, causing acidity of the blood. This leads to diabetic ketoacidosis. When severe, this can lead to diabetic coma, swelling of the brain and even death.

The published evidence of complications and deaths for those with type 1 diabetes combined with disordered eating is staggering. One report indicates that the mortality rate is three times the mortality rate of those with diabetes alone. The average life span of those who restrict insulin is 13 years less than those who don't restrict insulin routinely.

> *THE MORTALITY RATE FOR THOSE WITH DIABULIMIA TRIPLES COMPARED TO THOSE WHO JUST HAVE DIABETES.*

Consequence II: Blurred Vision and Diabetic Retinopathy (Eye Disease)

Marilyn, age 31:
"I skipped my insulin and ruined my eyesight. "

> *"When I was 10 years old I was diagnosed with type 1 diabetes. I did whatever I was supposed to until high school when I started to compare myself to other girls and felt pudgy. Then I made what I thought was a great discovery: If I didn't take as much insulin I didn't have to worry about what I ate and I could stay thin. For a few years, I let my A1c soar to 12. I cannot believe how many years I did this. As long as I looked good, that's all I cared about.*
>
> *Then one day I was driving along going to work, heading down the freeway, and suddenly I could not see the other cars on the freeway clearly. They were just kind of like blurred shapes whizzing by all around me, and the signs were all out of focus, and I was scared to death.*
>
> *I went to an ophthalmologist and he gave me the diagnosis: I had retinopathy. I got it from having such high blood sugar for so long. By the time I was 30 years old, I was legally blind. No more driving, no more working on the computer. Everything in my life has changed. If I had only known what I was doing to myself I would have asked for help sooner."*

When the blood glucose rapidly changes from normal to high, the eye lenses swell (osmotic change) causing blurring of vision. This condition is transient, often lasting 20-30 minutes. It is reversible as long as the blood glucose stabilizes to normal range; although rarely, permanent cataracts (opacities) may form in the lens.

Serious problems can occur from prolonged elevations of the blood glucose over years of diabetes. Prolonged elevations in blood glucose can affect the blood vessels at the back of the eye (diabetic retinopathy), which is the leading cause of blindness in the United States. Between 12,000 and 23,000 people lose their eyesight each year due to diabetic complications.

Blurred vision is reversible as long as blood glucose gets back under control in a short period of time.

However, if the blood glucose stays high over a number of years, the stages of diabetic retinopathy occur one after another:

Simple diabetic retinopathy:

Development of minute bubbles in the wall of a small blood vessel of retina (micro-aneurysms), usually non-vision-threatening.

Moderate diabetic retinopathy:

Blockage of blood flow in the vessels; swelling in the center of the retina (macula edema).

Advanced diabetic retinopathy:
Formation of abnormal, fragile blood vessels in the eye (neovascularization). These new, fragile vessels may bleed, causing loss of vision.

A 2008 study was done in a Japanese women's medical center to determine the length of time it takes for people with type 1 diabetes to develop retinopathy after diabetes onset. In this study it took an average of 11.5 years for simple retinopathy to develop, and 15.9 years for advanced retinopathy to develop.

However, when type 1 diabetes occurred in combination with eating disorders, it took an average of only 3.4 years to develop simple retinopathy, and 7.6 years to develop advanced retinopathy.

Consequence III: Diabetic Neuropathy (Nerve Damage) and Limb Amputation

Some develop mild to severe nervous system damage after 20 to 30 years of diabetes. This may include impaired sensation or pain in the feet or hands; slowed digestion of food in the stomach; carpal tunnel syndrome or other nerve problems.

Between three and five people per 1000 with diabetes suffer from gangrene, which is the death of tissues leading to lower-limb amputations. This occurs because continual exposure to high blood glucose causes damage to the nerves in the body. The longer this continues, and the higher the glucose values, the grater the damage to the nerves.

Remember Mary's story? She cried out: *"Now I can hardly walk, some of my toes have turned purple and some are completely black. I was told I would lose my feet and could possibly lose my legs as well. I am only 28."*

> *MARY'S PERIPHERAL NEUROPATHY CAUSED NERVE DAMAGE, NUMBNESS, AND ULTIMATELY GANGRENE AND AMPUTATIONS.*

Diabetic neuropathy (the damage of nerves) is classified into four types. One may suffer from only one or a combination of these types depending on the blood glucose control.

Peripheral neuropathy affects the peripheral nervous system, which is the network of nerves used for all movements (motor nerves) and sensations (sensory nerves). The symptoms of nerve damage include tingling, numbness (often becomes permanent), burning (especially in the evening) and pain. Lower extremities such as feet and legs are most affected.

Diabetic autonomic neuropathy affects the and regulates involunt such as the digestive s urinary system, blood heart and glands. The symptoms may inc bloating, feeling full ev small meals, diarrhea, constipation, heartbur incontinence (leaking u impotence, nausea and vomiting.

Proximal neuropathy (nearer to the center of the body) causes pain in the thighs, hips, or buttocks; it can also lead to weakness in the legs.

Focal (local area) neuropathy affects one nerve or one group of nerves, resulting in sudden pain or weakness of that area. Any nerve in the body may be affected, causing symptoms such as severe pain in the lower back or leg, paralysis on one side of the face, or weakness of an eye muscle causing double vision.

Kevin, age 34:
"I may be in a wheelchair for the rest of my life."

"I have had type 1 diabetes for almost 22 years now. I was on the track team in high school; keeping myself "light" to run fast was my priority. For eight of those years, I didn't take much insulin, just enough to "get by." Well, I certainly didn't "get by" with anything as it turns out. What I got are big time problems with my feet. I can no longer jog or play golf -- now it hurts just to walk.

I get all these terrible sharp pains now and they are getting worse. It is impossible to function well when you're in pain and I am not functioning well, that's for sure. At night is when the pain is almost unbearable. I can barely stand to walk upstairs to the bedroom. I am 34 years old. I desperately hope I can get some help before I am wheelchair-bound for the rest of my life."

This painful peripheral neuropathy was found in 37.5 percent of the eating-disordered patients with diabetes. According to one report the painful sensation coincides with the peak of weight loss due to high blood glucose.

Consequence IV: Diabetic Nephropathy (Kidney Disease) and Dialysis

In order to understand the development of diabetic kidney disease it is important to understand how the kidneys work. The kidneys are a pair of bean-shaped organs that sit below the ribs in the back of the torso. Each kidney is made up of over a million nephrons, a network of small tubes. Each nephron contains a glomerulus that is encapsulated by hundreds of blood vessels.

Healthy kidneys act like a filter to make sure the right amount of waste and fluids are removed; they keep the acid-base and electrolytes in balance; regulate blood pressure; and produce hormones. Kidneys filter 180 liters of blood and excrete two liters of urine daily.

The waste products in the blood include urea, uric acid and nitrogen (derived from protein) products. If these products accumulate in the blood they can lead to neurological impairment; i.e., alteration of mental status due to brain damage (encephalopathy); coma and even death.

Hyperglycemia can damage the structures of glomeruli, causing them to thicken and become scarred. Slowly, over time, more and more of the glomeruli are destroyed. The kidney structures begin to leak protein (albumin) which passes into the urine.

The presence of a small amount of protein in the urine is called micoralbuminuria. A normal microalbumin urine test is less than 30mg/dL. Thirty to 300 mg/dL indicates early kidney disease (microalbuminuria) and more than 300 mg/dL indicates more advanced kidney disease (macroalbuminuria).

Some of the symptoms of diabetic kidney disease are: delayed onset of puberty and growth retardation in adolescence; headache, nausea, vomiting, fatigue; high blood pressure; swelling around the eyes, the lower extremities and legs; and shortness of breath. When the kidney function drops below 15 percent, dialysis is inevitable. In some severe cases, a kidney transplant is necessary to sustain life.

The Japan study indicated that it could take only 6.6 years for individuals with type 1 diabetes to develop diabetic nephropathy if practicing insulin omission, rather than an average of 15.1 years for those without eating disorders.

Melissa, age 49:
"I am in kidney failure because of diabulimia."

"I used to be athletic. I was on the soccer team and swim team in junior high and high school. I have had diabetes as long as I can remember, since the age of four. I learned to take the right amount of insulin so I wouldn't feel tired in order to perform well. I kept my A1c around 7 to 8% -- my parents and my doctors were pleased with that.

When I went to college, I gained the "freshman 15" pounds the first year, plus more during the next three years because I was no longer playing sports. I relied on take out meals and fast food since Mom wasn't there making sure I ate right. Also I went out drinking with my friends pretty frequently. I thought I could prevent the weight gain if I didn't take all my insulin.

I kept it up after I was married, and didn't even share this "secret" with my husband. I knew he would ask me to get help if I told him. Now here I am, twenty seven years later at age 49 and I am in complete kidney failure. I have to be on dialysis. A machine is keeping me alive! How did this happen? "

AT AGE 49 MELISSA IS ON DIALYSIS BECAUSE OF INSULIN OMISSION.

Chapter 7

ONGOING TREATMENT
Why Every Discipline Is Important;
How and Where to Find the Best Care

Diabulimia is a deadly serious dual condition. For individuals to successfully recover requires a group effort. They must work with the entire professional team; each member has a crucial role to play. The team should include: Endocrinologist/diabetologist, diabetes nurse educator, psychologist/social worker, psychiatrist and registered dietitian. A multidisciplinary team approach to treatment is considered the standard of care.

Endocrinologists/Diabetologists and Diabetes Nurse Educators

For those who have yet to find an endocrinologist, the first step is to consult your nearest medical center and make an appointment with a diabetes clinic. Also, there are several websites providing lists of endocrinologists on the internet. For the pediatric population, there is the Pediatric Endocrine Society (http://www.lwpes.org/patientsFamilies/patientsandfamilies.cfm). For adults there is the American Association of Clinical Endocrinologists (www.aace.com). A diabetes clinic specializing in type 1 diabetes is the best place to start.

Many people think their medical visits will only entail a simple insulin adjustment. The truth is that it takes a thorough evaluation and ongoing follow-up to detect and prevent most complications. There may not be any symptoms in the early stages of complications and therefore, screening tests are important. Early detection is really the key since most complications are not reversible in advanced stages when symptoms may be present.

An endocrinologist will check for these things during the first visit:

- Full medical history including medications

- Review of symptoms

- Full physical examination including vital signs, eye exam, thyroid exam

- Laboratory measurements, such as hemoglobin A1c, tests for microalbuminuria, and celiac disease if indicated.

- Referral to other specialists as needed, such as eye (retinal) specialists.

The endocrinologists will be looking for danger signs:

- Tingling sensations, numbness or pain in the extremities

- Bloated stomach

- Blurred vision

- High blood pressure

- Slightly swollen feet or puffy eyelids

- Diminished reflexes and/or loss of sensation on feet

- Lesions on the legs

> *IF DANGER SIGNS ARE ADDRESSED RIGHT AWAY, THE PROBLEMS CAN OFTEN BE REVERSED OR KEPT FROM PROGRESSING TO MORE ADVANCED STAGES*

Jodie, age 42:
"I passed out in my cubicle at work and the next thing I knew I was
going on dialysis."

"I thought as long as I kept taking some insulin, I didn't have to bother going back to the doctor all the time. One day at work my head hurt so badly I thought I was having a stroke. I passed out before I could even call for help. The next thing I knew I woke up in a hospital room and a kidney doctor was telling me how dialysis works.

The kidney doctor explained that if I had just been seeing an endocrinologist regularly he would have picked up on my symptoms: blood pressure going up, protein in the urine, headache... I sure wish I had paid attention to all that when it was still reversible. It's too late to prevent dialysis now. And I'm only 42."

JODIE'S SYMPTOMS INDICATED SHE WAS IN DANGER. SHE IGNORED THEM, DID NOT SEE AN ENDOCRINOLOGIST, AND SUFFERED KIDNEY FAILURE.

An endocrinology team will administer tests, take readings and measurements, do screenings initially, and then follow up to monitor changes and trends quarterly or periodically.

To prevent permanent damage, screen for complications related to diabetes at regular intervals, according to this standard of care.

- **Ophthalmologic(eyes) Evaluation:** Start at the age of ten years and when diabetes duration is three to five years.

- **Microalbuminuria (protein in the urine) Assessment:** Start at ten years of age and when diabetes duration is five years.

- **Lipid Profile:** These screenings should start at two years of age if there is a positive or unknown family history of heart disease. If the family history is negative, annual lipid profiling should begin at puberty.

- **Celiac and Adrenal Antibodies, TSH Tests:** Test annually or every other year. If symptoms or poor growth is noted, test more frequently.

- **Depression Screenings:** Begin at ten years of age.

Psychotherapists

Finding a psychotherapist who treats both eating disorders and chronic illness may be challenging. One good option is to work with a therapist who is already a team member of a diabetes clinic. Also, the endocrinologist may be able to give referrals to psychotherapists who work closely with them. There are multiple commercial websites listing psychotherapists who specialize in eating disorders. Individuals and families must be sure to ask if the psychotherapist is willing to work closely with a diabetes team.

Prior to scheduling an appointment, individuals and families may **interview psychotherapists on the phone,** asking a few simple and clarifying questions, such as:

- *Do you treat eating disorders? If so, for how many years?*

- *What percentage of your practice involves eating disorders?*

- *Are you comfortable treating someone with type 1 diabetes?*

- *Have you treated cases of diabulimia?*

- *Are you willing to learn more about diabetes with eating disorders?*

- *Will you work with my diabetes team closely?*

Psychological Treatment

Weekly or bi-weekly appointments with a mental health professional are crucial for the recovery of diabulimia (ED-DMT1). Many families feel ashamed or embarrassed to think that their loved ones have any kind of mental health problem, so they are reluctant to seek help for them. Many individuals too, deny the psychological side of their illness. They prefer to avoid dealing with their emotions and actions.

Brenda, age 15:
"My parents refused to take me back to the psychotherapist."

"My Mom told the doctor "No way does she need a shrink!" Of course, my parents didn't really know how much insulin I took. They thought if the endocrinologist would just prescribe the "right dose" of insulin, and if the dietitian would just teach me the "correct information" everything would be fine.

They're OK with their daughter having diabetes, but they're not OK with me having an eating disorder. They think you must have some sort of mental problem if you have to see a therapist. We went once, and my parents said it was a total waste of time. We never went back. So I still haven't really talked about my "problem".

> WHEN FAMILIES REJECT PSYCHOLOGICAL TREATMENT, RECOVERY FROM DIABULIMIA CAN BE DELAYED.

To address the issues of diabulimia there are several psychological approaches, often combined. The most common ones are:

- **Cognitive Behavioral Therapy** (CBT)- Enhanced for Eating Disorders -- emphasizes the thinking, and the actions of reintroduction of regular eating, weight exposure, and treating body image concerns.

- **Dialectical Behavioral Therapy** (DBT) is a treatment that combines techniques of CBT and emotional regulation. It is often provided in a group format.

- **Family-Based Therapy** (FBT) enlists the family as a resource to help their child through behavioral management of symptoms. This is an especially helpful treatment for children and adolescents with diabulimia.

All the treatments have the same purpose: To help individuals change destructive and unhealthy behavior by first recognizing the thinking behind it, then learning how to replace it. Also, a distorted perception of body image is common in eating disorders and is often addressed cognitively. In addition, the family's way of perceiving and dealing with the maladaptive behavior may be counterproductive, and may even inadvertently reinforce it. That is one reason why family therapy is crucial, especially for adolescents.

Individuals with diabulimia may also be evaluated by a psychiatrist for the need for psychiatric medications. Medications for anxiety and mood disorders may also have a role in the treatment plan.

Registered Dietitians

It is extremely important to work with a dietitian who has a great passion for treating individuals with eating disorders. The RD (registered dietitian) must not only understand diabetes but also be skillful in managing blood glucose patterns associated with an insulin regimen or food intake.

Make sure to look for an RD who is actively working with a diabetes team either in the hospital or in a diabetes clinic. A dietitian with a CDE certification (certified diabetes educator) is a plus. Ideally, individuals should work with a dietitian who is a member of the diabetes team, as opposed to getting referrals to outside dietitians who may be more familiar with type 2 diabetes treatments.

There are quite a few commercial and non-profit organizations with websites listing dietitians who treat eating disorders. However, most of these organizations require membership fees, which lower the percentage of dietitians willing to join. The official website of the American Dietetic Association, www.eatright.org, provides a comprehensive listing of dietitians, arranged by locations. People should look for one nearby and ask some questions when calling:

- *In your practice, what percentage of your clients has eating disorders and what percentage has diabetes?*

- *Do many of your clients with diabetes have type 1, or are the majority of them type 2?*

- *How many cases of diabulimia have you treated? Over 20?10?*

Medical Nutrition Therapy

The role of dietitians in treating individuals with diabulimia can never be over emphasized. Nutritional education is the key. Many of these clients have tried and failed with various weight loss diets which are not safe for them. Chapter 8, Nutrition and Diabulimia, addresses the functions of major nutrients in association with diabetes and eating disorders. It contains nutrition guides for those with diabulimia, an alternative to counting carbohydrates, meal plans and information on common botanical products.

WEIGHT MEASUREMENT –
THE PROS AND CONS OF REVEALING BODY WEIGHT

In the early stage of medical nutrition therapy, weekly weight checks and nutrition appointments are recommended. This does not necessarily mean the individual must be made aware of weekly weight results. The dietitian should discuss this issue with the treatment team, particularly the psychotherapist and family therapist, to work out the best approach for revealing (or not revealing) a client's weight.

Some individuals become obsessed with body weight. They may further restrict food intake or decrease insulin if they see their weight climbing. In such cases it is better to weigh clients without revealing the numbers. On the other hand, some may feel anxious not knowing what the scales show, and falsely assume they have gained weight. This may lead to further attempts to find inappropriate ways to lose weight. Also, they may be weighing obsessively at home and already be determined to thwart   treatment for fear of weight gain. In that case, the numbers on the scale need to be monitored and discussed openly. The dietitian must be ready to work with such clients closely.

RESOURCES

Many non-profit organizations provide educational materials and information of health personnel in various disciplines.

DIABETES

- AADE: American Association of Diabetes Educators

  www.diabeteseducator.org

- AACE: American Association of Clinical Endocrinologists

  www.aace.com

- ADA: American Diabetes Association

  www.diabetes.org

- Children with Diabetes

  www.childrenwithdiabetes.com

- The Diabetes Society

  www.diabetessociety.org

- Diabetes Youth Foundation

  www.dyf.org

- International Diabetes Federation

  www.idf.org

- JDRF: Juvenile Diabetes Research Foundation

  www.jdrf.org

- NDEI: National Diabetes Education Initiative

  www.ndei.org

- NDEP: National Diabetes Education Program

  www.ndep.nih.gov

- Pediatric Endocrine Society
  http://www.lwpes.org/patientsFamilies/patientsandfamilies.cfm

NUTRITION

- ADA: American Dietetic Association

  www.eatright.org

- ASN: American Society for Nutrition

  www.nutrition.org

- USDA Food Pyramid and nutrition education information

  www.mypyramid.gov

EATING DISORDERS

- AED: Academy for Eating Disorders
  www.aedweb.org

- ANAD: Association of Anorexia Nervosa & Associated Disorders
  www.anad.org

- Anna Westin Foundation
  www.annawestinfoundation.org

Bulimia Nervosa Resource Guide
www. bulimiaguide.org

EDA: Eating Disorders Anonymous
www.eatingdisordersanonymous.org

Eating Disorders Coalition for Research, Policy & Action
www.eatingdisorderscoalition.com

EDIN: Eating Disorders Information Network
www.edin-ga.org

EDRC: Eating Disorders Resource Center

www.edrcsv.org

- FEAST: Family Empowered and Supporting Treatment of Eating Disorders

  www.feast-ed.org

- Kristen Watt Foundation

  www.kristenwattfoundation.org

- NEDA: National Eating Disorders Association
  www.NationalEatingDisorders.org

- National Eating Disorders Screening Program
  www.mentalhealthscreening.org

Chapter 8

NUTRITION AND DIABULIMIA

Individuals with eating disorders have misconceptions about food. They may deprive themselves of fats, carbohydrates or total calories in their obsession about losing weight. They think fats make you fat, carbohydrates make you gain weight, and the more you cut down on calories the thinner you'll be. Sensible eating that incorporates a healthy amount of fats, carbohydrates and protein may frighten them.

Yet, for those with type 1 diabetes, each of those nutrients is a necessity because it directly impacts blood glucose levels and body function. Susie down the street can go without certain nutrients for a time with few harmful effects. But if her friend Jane with type 1 diabetes tries it, her blood glucose will be unstable, and she may put herself in jeopardy.

Most existing nutritional information has emphasized either the importance of balanced eating for those with diabetes, or it has emphasized correcting the erratic eating patterns seen in eating disorders. Individuals with diabulimia desperately need guidance about both, but it has not been available until the publication of this book. With nowhere to turn, they go on making dangerous food choices. Dangerous because poor choices that are detrimental to the metabolism of blood glucose further contribute to the complications of type 1 diabetes. Complications, as this book has explained, that are dire, life-changing and even fatal.

This chapter on nutrition is crucial in that it deals with the way nutrients affect blood glucose and impact diabetes, while simultaneously dealing with educating those with eating disorders and correcting their dangerous misconceptions about food. The author's expertise and unique perspective as a registered dietician specializing in both eating disorders and diabetes lends credence to this vital information. Finally caregivers and families have access to all the pieces needed to solve the puzzle of nutrition related to diabulimia.

.Why Calories?

Asleep or awake, active or inactive, the body needs a constant supply of fuel (calories) just for basic daily functions. Even a body at rest burns approximately 1200 to 1600 calories per 24 hour period. That is the approximate Basal Metabolic Rate (BMR) for an average weight adult to keep the resting metabolism going. For a teenager who is growing, developing and going through puberty, the BMR could be even higher. When the body does not receive adequate calories for metabolism, it starts breaking down body cells and tissues (catabolism) as fuel. That is why a restricted diet is not recommended.

What does the body do with all those calories, even when it is at rest? These are just some of the ways calories are used every 24 hours:

Your heart beats	103,689 times
You use	7,000,000 brain cells
You breathe	23,040 times
You inhale	438 cubic feet of air
You move	750 major muscles
You perspire	1.43 pints of moisture
Your blood travels	168,000 miles
You speak	48,000 words
Your hail grows	0.1717 inches
Your nails grow	0.00046 inches
Your body digests	3.5 pounds of foods
Your body processes	2.9 pounds of liquids

On top of that, more calories are burned through household activities, school, work and exercise. Appropriate caloric intake for teenagers and adults is approximately 2000 to 2800 kcal depending on age, sex, body weight, individual metabolism and physical activities.

Why Protein?

Protein is the major building block of the body. It is the primary component of muscle tissue and is essential for the formation of all tissues, cells, blood, enzymes, antibodies and hormones. Every cell in the body, except those in the bile and urine, contains protein.

The average teenager and adult needs 0.8 -1.2 gram of protein per kilogram of body weight (one kilogram=2.2 pounds). In other words, a 120 pound person needs around 55 grams of protein daily. A sensible way to consume 55 grams of protein a day would be to eat four ounces of fish, fowl or meat; two to three servings of dairy; and a half cup of combined grains and legumes. Protein does not increase plasma glucose concentrations; combining protein with carbohydrates can prevent an upsurge in an individual's post-meal blood glucose.

> THE LIFE SPAN OF CELLS IS TWO TO THREE WEEKS. TO BUILD NEW CELLS, THE BODY NEEDS APPROXIMATELY 55 TO 75 GRAMS OF PROTEIN A DAY.

Protein is composed of chains of amino acids. Some amino acids can be synthesized in the body. However, nine of them can only come from food sources; these are called the essential amino acids. All animal proteins such as meats, poultry, fish, eggs, and dairy products contain complete protein; i.e., all nine essential amino acids are present. Incomplete plant proteins such as soy, nuts, lentils and legumes contain only some of the nine essential amino acids.

Amino Acids Food Sources

	Lysine	Isoleucine	Tryptophan	Methionine	Cystine
Legumes Soybeans, lentils, peas, black-eyed peas, chickpeas, peanuts	yes	yes			
Grains Rice, wheat, oats, corn, barley, rye, buckwheat			yes	yes	yes
Seeds and nuts Sesame, sunflower, pine nuts, pecans			yes	yes	yes
Egg, milk, Meats, Fish	yes	yes	yes	yes	yes

Complete Protein Pairings and Examples

Pairing	Examples
Legumes with Grains	Beans and tortillas
	Hummus with pita bread
	Chickpeas and rice
	Black-eyed peas and rice
	Peanut butter sandwich
Legumes with Seeds	Hummus
Grains with Dairy/Eggs	Macaroni and cheese
	Oatmeal with milk
	Pizza
	Rice pudding
	Egg salad sandwich
Nuts/Seeds with Dairy	Yogurt with nuts and/or seeds
Dairy/Eggs with Vegetables	Eggplant parmesan
	Vegetable omelet
	Vegetable quiche

Why Fats?

The benefits of fats in the diet cannot be ignored. Without them, brain tissues could be damaged, growth in height could be stunted, and puberty development could be delayed. Not only that, many vitamins are fat-soluble, such as A, D, E, and K, all of which rely on fats to transport them into the cells. Without fats, vitamin A, D, E or K deficiency becomes inevitable. Current research studies have paid a great deal of attention to the role of essential fatty acids (such as omega-3 or omega-6 fatty acids) in retinal development during infancy, as well as the role of essential fatty acids in heart disease prevention, and the protection of inflammation.

Foods high in fat have a unique effect on blood sugar. While fat does not raise glucose levels, it slows the absorption of carbohydrates consumed in the same meal. It delays the peak glycemic response, thus prolonging steady blood glucose levels for individuals with type 1 diabetes.

Individuals with eating disorders often avoid fats in their diet. Their misconception is that eating fats makes them fat. It's the total amount of calories, not the number of fat grams that moves body weight up or down. Appropriate fat intake (both plant and animal fats) should equal 20 to 35 percent of the total daily calories consumed, or 50 to100 grams of fat daily. Daily optimal essential fatty acids (such as omega-3) intake is one gram a day or 6 to 8 grams a week.

Food Sources of Omega 3 Fatty Acids

Food	Portion Size	Amount of Omega 3 FA (g)
Fish		
Bluefish, fresh or frozen	4 oz.	1.7
Cod, fresh and frozen	4 oz.	0.6
Crab, soft shell, cooked	4 oz.	0.6
Lobster, cooked	4 oz.	0.1
Mackerel, canned	4 oz.	2.2
Salmon, canned	4 oz.	2.2
Salmon, cold water, fresh and frozen	4 oz.	1.7
Sardines, canned in oil	4 oz.	1.8
Scallops, Maine, fresh, frozen	4 oz.	0.5
Smelt, rainbow	4 oz.	0.5
Swordfish, fresh, frozen	4 oz.	1.7
Tuna, canned in water	4 oz.	0.3
Tuna, canned in oil	4 oz.	0.2
Oils		

Canola oil	1 Tbsp.	1.3
Cod liver oil	1 Tbsp.	2.8
Flax seed oil	1 Tbsp.	6.9
Olive oil	1 Tbsp.	0.1
Sardine oil	1 Tbsp.	3.7
Soybean oil	1 Tbsp.	0.9
Walnut oil	1 Tbsp.	1.4
Legumes, seeds, nuts, grains		
Almonds, dry roasted	1 oz.	0
Flax seeds	1 oz.	1.8
Pecans, dry roasted	1 oz.	0.3
Pistachios, roasted	1 oz.	0.1
Poppy seeds	1 oz.	0.1
Pumpkin seeds, shelled	1 oz.	0.1
Soybeans, dried, cooked	½ cup	0.5
Tofu, regular	4 oz.	0.3
Walnuts	1 oz.	2.6

Why Carbohydrates?

Carbohydrate is broken down into glucose when it is digested; insulin then serves as a key allowing glucose to enter the cells. Glucose is the fuel for the body and it is the absolute energy source of the brain and nerve system.

Current studies indicate that the same number of carbohydrates in meals causes the same glucose response regardless of whether the carbohydrate source is a simple sugar or a starch. However, when the same amount of carbohydrate is eaten at a meal in addition to protein and fat, the glucose response differs. Adding protein and fat to the carbohydrate prevents a spike in the post-meal blood glucose level. For instance: having cereal with milk, toast with peanut butter, fruit with yogurt, or pancakes with eggs for breakfast are all good examples of protein, fat and carbohydrate combinations.

Appropriate carbohydrates are: 35 to 50 grams for breakfast; 45 to 60 grams for lunch; 60 to 80 grams for dinner; and 5 to 30 grams for snacks, (total daily carbohydrates about 130 to 230 grams) depending on age and physical activity levels.

The benefits of fiber

Fiber is extremely beneficial to the body. Fiber keeps bowel movements regular and may reduce the risk of colon problems. Some studies indicated that adequate fiber intake may reduce low density lipoprotein-cholesterol, LDL (the bad cholesterol) and enhance the high density lipoprotein-cholesterol, HDL (the good cholesterol).

The ideal daily fiber intake is 25 to 35 grams, which can easily be obtained from three servings of fruit, one cup of vegetables and half a cup of whole grains.

The danger of a low carbohydrate diet

The American Diabetic Association (ADA) does not recommend a daily carbohydrate intake below 130 grams for teens and adults. For individuals with diabetes, the ADA advises against low carbohydrate diets under any circumstances.

A low carbohydrate diet could possibly lead to initial weight reduction from loss of fluid. However, if the weight loss is sustained it is because of the reduction of total calories. Studies of those who are on a low carbohydrate diet for over six months indicated higher levels of low density lipoprotein-cholesterol (LDL), the bad cholesterol, are present.

For those with diabetes, a low carbohydrate diet is particularly dangerous because the low blood glucose levels may lead to hypoglycemic symptoms such as shaking, sweating, and confusion and could even lead to seizure, coma and unconsciousness.

Gloria, age 17:
"My low carb diet led to a seizure."

"One night when I was studying for my finals I started to shake like crazy. For the past few days, I felt really tired but I thought it was just because I was studying so hard and not sleeping enough. My friend and I had been on a low carbohydrate diet. I thought it was great because her sister lost 10 pounds in three weeks doing low carb. So I ate lots of chicken and tons of salads. It seemed so healthy. I didn't have to take much insulin because most of what I ate was "free" foods. My blood sugar was 82 when I checked the day before and I remember my father telling me how well I was doing. But by the next night, he was frantically calling 911 because he thought I was having a seizure."

> *GLORIA LEARNED THAT HAVING TYPE 1 DIABETES MEANS CARBOHYDRATES ARE A NECESSITY.*

Why Vitamins and Minerals?

Fat-soluble vitamins

Vitamins A, D, E, and K are fat-soluble vitamins, which require fats to transport them to the cells. When more are taken than needed, they are stored in the liver, above safe upper limits, which can be toxic.

Fat Soluble Vitamin	Why You Need Them	Recommended Amount* (DRI**)	Food Sources
Vitamin A	Protects against night blindness; helps maintain normal vision; aids in immune system	980-2970 IU Safe upper limit: 9240-9900 IU	Carrots, organ meats, sweet potatoes, eggs, leafy green vegetables, fortified milk
Vitamin D	Aids calcium absorption and maintains normal blood level of calcium and phosphorus; provides bone health	600 IU Safe upper limit: 2000 IU	Fortified milk, fish oil, cod liver oil, organ meats
Vitamin E	Protects against cell oxidation or radical damage, is an antioxidant and promotes strong immunity	16-22 IU Safe upper limit: 895-1492 IU	Vegetable oil, seeds, wheat germ, nuts, legumes, eggs
Vitamin K	Assists in clotting of blood	60-120 mcg	Dark, leafy, green vegetables, eggs

*Amounts are for ages 11 and above and vary according to the specific age. **
Dietary Reference Intakes, Food and Nutrition Board, Institute of Medicine, National Academics Press, Washington DC, 2010.

Water-soluble vitamins

The water-soluble vitamins include vitamins C and B complex: B_1 (thiamin), B_2 (riboflavin), niacin, B_6, and B_{12}. Excess amounts are excreted via the kidneys to the urine and are not toxic.

Water-Soluble Vitamin	Why You Need Them	Recommended Amount* (DRI**)	Food Sources
Vitamin B_1 (Thiamin)	Plays an essential role in metabolizing carbohydrates; promote healthy nerve system	0.9 – 1.2 mg	Yeast, liver and grains
Vitamin B_2 (Riboflavin)	Assists in metabolizing carbohydrates, amino acids, and lipids; helps with utilization of energy; Supports antioxidants	0.9-1.3 mg	Dairy products, organ meats, fortified cereals, meats, eggs
Niacin	Used as a co-enzyme in the pathway of carbohydrates, amino acids, and fatty acids metabolism; assists in energy utilization	12-16 mg	Meats, fortified cereals, grains, tuna, eggs

Vitamin B$_6$	Assists in metabolizing amino acids	1.0-1.3 mg	Meats, grains, fortified cereals, seeds, potato, banana
Vitamin B$_{12}$	Assists in metabolizing all cells, especially in the gastrointestinal tract, bone marrow, and never system	1.8-2.4 mg	Organ meats, meats, seafood, dairy products ***This vitamin can only be obtained from animal food sources. Strict vegetarians need to take vitamin B$_{12}$ supplements.**
Vitamin C	Helps with formation of collagen; aides immune system; helps iron absorption	45 – 90 mg	Fruits and vegetables

*Amounts are for ages 11 and above and vary according to the specific age.

** Dietary Reference Intakes, Food and Nutrition Board, Institute of Medicine, National Academics Press, Washington DC, 2010.

Minerals

Mineral	Why You Need Them	Recommended Amount* (DRI**)	Food Sources
Calcium	Promotes healthy bones and teeth: assists in blood clotting; aids in muscles contraction and relaxation	1000 – 1300 mg	Dairy products, canned sardines, dry fish with bone, dark, green leafy vegetables, tofu
Chromium	Helps metabolize carbohydrates and may enhance the effectiveness of insulin	25-35 mcg	Brewer's yeast, broccoli, red meats, eggs, seafood
Copper	Helps form red blood cells, metabolism of iron, and maintenance of blood vessels	700 – 900 mcg	Oysters, shellfish, nuts, organ meats, legumes, green, leafy vegetables
Iodine	Helps produce thyroxin, which regulates thyroid function	120-150 mcg	Seafood, seaweed, iodized salt
Iron	Helps form	8-18 mg	**Heme iron food**

	hemoglobin, the substance in blood that carries oxygen through the body		**sources (better absorption):** red meats, organ meats, eggs, oysters **Non-heme sources:** dark, leafy greens, lentils, dried fruits, iron-fortified cereals
Magnesium	Maintains normal muscle and nerve function; keeps heart rhythm steady; supports immune system and healthy bones	240 – 420 mg	Seafood, nuts, whole grains, green vegetables, lentils, milk products
Potassium	Helps maintain fluid balance; regulates heart rhythm and muscle contractions	2000+ mg	Bananas, oranges, tomato, dairy products, meats, legumes
Phosphorus	Forms structure of bones, teeth, cell membranes, and DNA; transports energy as a coenzyme in cells	700 – 1250 mg	Meats, dairy products, eggs, seafood, whole grains

| Selenium | Prevents radical damage to cells; vital to immune system function as antioxidant | 40-55 mcg | Nuts, seeds, seafood, meats, eggs, grains, mushrooms, onions |
| Zinc | Promotes growth, cell reproduction, and repair; helps with immune function | 8-11 mg | Seafood, fortified cereals, seeds, meats, nuts, eggs |

*Amounts are for ages 11 and above and vary according to the specific age.
** Dietary Reference Intakes, Food and Nutrition Board, Institute of Medicine, National Academics Press, Washington DC, 2010.

When people receive adequate vitamins and minerals from their food sources, there is no evidence that vitamin and mineral supplementation is beneficial. Routine supplementation of antioxidants such as vitamins C, E or selenium is not advised. Chromium supplementation has been studied for its potential influence on glycemic index and insulin resistance. However, current studies do not conclusively demonstrate efficacy; therefore, the American Diabetic Association does not recommend chromium supplementation. Individuals on calorie-restricted diets, as well as pregnant and lactating women, elderly individuals and strict vegetarians may have a need for vitamin and mineral supplements.

IF AT ALL POSSIBLE, OBTAIN VITAMINS AND MINERALS FROM FOOD SOURCES, NOT SUPPLEMENTS.

Nutrition Guidelines for Those with Diabulimia

1. Count Carbohydrates

A 2002 study in Great Britain indicated that HbA1c levels were lower by 1 percent when individuals with type 1 diabetes were taught to adjust insulin per planned carbohydrate intake. The American Diabetic Association has recommended that monitoring total grams of carbohydrate, whether by carbohydrate counting or by using the exchange system, is the standard for medical nutrition therapy for those with type 1 diabetes.

2. Use Proper Portions

Check this chart to find portion sizes for different foods that equal 15 grams of carbohydrates.

FOOD	PORTION SIZE (Equal to 15 grams of carbohydrate)
Fruits (includes core, skin, seeds, and rind)	
Apple, small	1 (4 oz.)
Applesauce, unsweetened	½ cup
Banana, extra small	1 (4 oz.)
Blackberries	¾ cup
Blueberries	¾ cup
Cantaloupe, small	1 cup cubed
Cherries, sweet, fresh	12

Dried fruits	2 Tbsp.
Fruit cocktail	½ cup
Grapefruit, large	½
Grapes, small	17
Honeydew melon	1 slice or 1 cup cubed
Kiwi	1
Mango, small	½ fruit
Nectarine, small	1
Orange, small	1
Peaches, fresh, large	1
Pineapple, fresh	¾ cup
Plums, small	2
Strawberries	1 ¼ cup whole berries
Watermelon	1 ¼ cups cubed
Starches: Cereals, Grains, Breads, Beans	
Animal crackers	8
Bagel, large	¼ (1 oz.)
Baked beans	1/3 cup
Beans, cooked (black, garbanzo, kidney, lima, navy, pinto, white)	½ cup

Bread, white, whole grain, rye	1 slice
Crackers, round-butter type	6
Cereal, bran	½ cup
Cereal, cooked (oats, oatmeal)	½ cup
Cornbread	1 ¾ inch cube
Couscous	1/3 cup
English muffin	½
Graham cracker, 2 ½ - inch square	3
Granola	¼ cup
Hamburger or hot dog bun	½ (1 oz.)
Lentils, cooked (brown, green, yellow)	½ cup
Naan, 8 inches by 2 inches	1/4
Pancake (4 in. across, ¼ in. thick)	1
Pasta, cooked	1/3 cup
Peas, cooked (black-eyed, split)	½ cup
Popcorn	3 cups
Rice, white or brown, cooked	1/3 cup

Rice cakes, 4 inches across	2
Roll, plain, small	1
Taco shell, 5 inches across	2
Tortilla, corn, 6 inches across	1
Tortilla, flour, 6 inches across	1
Waffle, 4-inch square	1
Starchy Vegetables	
Corn, large cob	½ cup or ½ cob
Mixed vegetables with corn, peas, or pasta	1 cup
Peas, green	½ cup
Potato, baked	½ medium
Potato, mashed	½ cup
Potato, French fried	1 cup
Spaghetti	½ cup
Squash, winter (acorn, butternut)	1 cup
Yam, sweet potato, plain	½ cup
Dairy	
Milk, fat-free or low-fat (buttermilk, acidophilus milk, Lactaid)	1 cup

Yogurt, fat-free	6 oz.
Yogurt, reduced-fat	6 oz.

Choose Your Foods: Exchange Lists for Diabetes
American Diabetes Association & American Dietetic Association

3. Select "Free Foods" Wisely

Foods that are low in carbohydrates are referred to as free foods. However, some free foods are high in cholesterol, fats or calories. Check this chart to see which free foods are also wise choices in terms of calories.

Free Foods

Food group	Lower calorie	Higher calorie
Protein	Chicken	Cheese
	Cottage cheese	Nuts
	Egg	Peanut butter
	Fish	Pork
	Tofu	Steak
	Tuna	
	Turkey	
	Seafood	
Vegetables	All non-starchy vegetables	
Fats		Avocado

		Bagel Spread
		Butter
		Cream
		Cream cheese
		Margarine
		Oil
		Salad dressings
		Whipped cream

4. Choose a Healthy Low Carb Snack

Minimal Carbohydrate Snacks
Celery sticks with ½ Tbsp peanut butter
Cottage cheese
Hard boiled egg
Non-starchy vegetables
Nuts (1 oz. or about 8 pieces)
Popcorn (1 cup or less)
Salads (with minimal mayonnaise)
Chicken
Egg

Tofu

Tuna

Sugar-free Jell-O

Turkey slices

Vegetable soup

Snacks containing approx. 15 grams of carbohydrate

½ cup cottage cheese with ½ cup unsweetened canned fruit

½ meat sandwich

½ cup sugar-free pudding

1 slice of cheese with 7 saltine crackers

2 rice crackers with ½ Tbsp peanut butter

3 cups popcorn

6 oz. light plain yogurt

5. Read Nutrition Facts on Labels

Food labels show the number of carbohydrates for each serving of a particular food. This makes it easy to keep track of carbohydrates consumed. However, pay attention to the serving size shown. For instance the nutrition panel for canned kidney beans lists one serving as ½ cup, double the amount of carbohydrates when consuming the contents of the entire can; i.e., one cup.

Nutrition Facts

Kidney beans canned 1 cup, 8 oz

Serving size ½ cup

Amount per serving

Calories 108   Calories from Fat 7

	% Daily Value
Total Fat 1g	1%
Saturated Fat 0g	0%
Trans Fat 0g	
Cholesterol 0mg	0%
Sodium 380mg	16%
Total Carbohydrates 20g	7%
Dietary Fiber 7g	26
Sugars 3g	
Protein 6g	

Vitamin A 0%   Vitamin C 2%

If you don't have the food wrapper or container handy to check the label, you can look up most foods on one of the websites that provide nutritional information, such as www.NutritionData.self.com, and www.CalorieKing.com.

6. Stay in Healthy Carbohydrate, Fat and Protein Ranges

Having a balanced meal with healthy amount of carbohydrates, protein and fats, and spacing carbohydrates evenly throughout the day can also improve post-meal blood glucose control. Here are general guidelines:

45% TO 65% OF CALORIES EATEN SHOULD COME FROM **CARBOHYDRATES**.

10% TO 35% OF CALORIES EATEN SHOULD COME FROM **PROTEIN**.

20% TO 35% OF CALORIES EATEN SHOULD COME FROM FAT.

One good reference is: www.mypyrimad.gov for a healthy meal plan.

A Set Dose of Insulin per Meal Size

Counting carbohydrates can be troublesome and awkward in certain situations, and can trigger obsessive behavior in some with diabulimia. One alternative is to establish a set dose of insulin per meal size. This works very well for someone whose blood glucose is high (e.g. HbA1c over 10%). The priority is to bring the blood glucose down through the simplest means possible.

Jeff, age 15:

"It's bad enough to give myself insulin when I eat."

"My mom also wants me to make sure I count every gram of carbohydrates. Forget it; I just don't eat around her. At the clinic, they found out I haven't taken bolus insulin for a long time. I told them that I just didn't want to be bothered with counting carbohydrates even though I also tried to lose some weight. My nurse and dietitian came out with an idea I thought was doable:

When I eat a small meal	*I get 7 U insulin*
a big meal	*I get 15 U insulin*
a medium size meal	*I get 10 U insulin*

My dietitian helped me plan what different size meals were like for me."

Sample Meal Plans for Three Different Groups

I. For younger teens with moderate activities: suggesting 2-3 servings dairy, 5 oz protein, a cup of vegetables, 2-3 servings of fruit and 5-8 servings of grains and adequate essential fats. Meal plan provides total of 153 gram carbohydrates (CHO).

Breakfast: *CHO*

- 1 serving (1/2 cup) high fiber cereal   15 g

- 1 serving (1 cup) low fat milk   12 g

- One cup chopped melon   15 g

                                                                   Total= 42g

Lunch   *CHO*

- 2 oz deli sliced turkey

- 1 serving (1 oz.) string cheese

- 2 slices of whole wheat bread with mayo   24g

- One apple   15g

                                                          Total=   39 g

Snack: C*HO*

   • 2 cups popcorn   10 g

Dinner: *CHO*

   • 1 serving (3 oz) baked chicken

   • 2 servings (2/3 cup) brown rice   30 g

   • One cup roasted zucchini

   • 1 serving (3/4 cup) raspberries   15 g

   • 1 serving (1/2 cup) ice cream   17g

                                  Total=   62g

                   Total CHO for the day-=   153g

II. For older teens with moderate activities: suggesting 3 servings dairy, 5-7 oz protein, 1-2 cups of vegetables, 3 servings of fruit and 7-11 servings of grains and adequate essential fats. Meal plan provides total of 227 gram carbohydrates (CHO).

Breakfast: C*HO*

- 2 egg whites

- 1 English muffin   30 g

- 1 Tbsp jam   15 g

- 1 serving (1 cup) low fat milk   12 g

                                                      Total= 57 g

Lunch: C*HO*

- Turkey (2 oz.) and veggie sandwich:

    2 slices whole-wheat bread   30 g

    lettuce, tomato, onion

- 1 serving low or non-fat yogurt   12 g

- 1 small bag of baked chips   24 g

                                                      Total= 66 g

<u>Snack:</u>   <u>CHO</u>

- 1 serving (1/4 cup) dry fruits and nuts   17 g

- 1 serving (8 oz) low fat milk   12 g

Total = 29 g

<u>Dinner:</u>   <u>CHO</u>

- 2 servings meat balls (5 oz)

- 1 oz shredded cheese

- One cup green beans

- 3 servings (1.5 cup) whole wheat spaghetti   45 g

- 1 bowl of salad (lettuce, tomato, cucumber) and 2Tbs dressing

- One orange   15g

- 1 raisin oatmeal cookie   15g

Total = 75 g

Total CHO for the day= 227 g

III. For adults with moderate activities: suggesting 3 servings dairy, 2 cups vegetables, 3 servings of fruit, 6-10 servings of grains and adequate essential fats. This meal plan provides a total of 170 grams carbohydrates (CHO).

Breakfast: <u>CHO</u>

- 1 serving low-fat cottage cheese or yogurt   12 g

- 2 servings (1/2 cup) low-fat granola   30 g

- 1 small orange or half of grapefruit   15 g

                                                                         Total= 57 g

Lunch: <u>CHO</u>

- 1 serving (2 Tbsp) hummus

- 2 small whole-wheat pita bread   30 g

- 1 serving (1/2 cup) red pepper slices

- 1 serving strawberries (1 ¼ cup)   15 g

                                                                         Total= 45 g

<u>*Snack:*</u>   <u>*CHO*</u>

- 5 whole-wheat crackers   11 g

- 1 Tbsp of peanut butter

- 4 carrot sticks

<u>*Dinner:*</u>   <u>*CHO*</u>

- 1 serving ground turkey (3 oz)

- 1 serving taco shells (2 shells)   15 g

- 1 serving (1/2 cup)   lettuce and shredded carrot

- One serving (1/2 cup) refried beans   15 g

- One serving (6 oz) Greek yogurt   12 g

- A serving of fruit   15g

                                    Total= 57g

                        Total CHO for the day= 170g

Be Aware of the Side Effects of Herbal and Botanical Products

Curious about herbal supplements and their roles in decreasing blood glucose? Remember, not all of them are safe or effective. Scrutinize the following list of products and their side effects. Keep in mind, too, that these supplements and herbs can negatively interact with drugs commonly used for diabetes.

PRODUCT	SIDE EFFECTS	DRUG INTERACTIONS
Aloe	None reported	Possible hypoglycemia if combined with secretagogues; Intraoperative blood loss in surgery patients where sevoflurance was used
Banaba	None reported	Possible hypoglycemia if combined with secretagogues
Bilberry	Mild gastrointestinal distress; Skin rashes	None known
Bitter melon	Gastrointestinal discomfort; Hypoglycemic coma; Favism; Hemolytic anemia in persons with G6PDH deficiency; Contains known abortifacients; Seeds have produced vomiting, death in	Hypoglycemia when used with sulfonylureas

	children	
Caiapo	Constipation, gastrointestinal pain	Possible hypoglycemia if combined with secretagogues
Chromium	Related to excessive intake and include renal toxicity	May decrease blood glucose if used with secretagogues
Cinnamon	No side effects reported; may cause irritation or dermatitis if used topically	May decrease blood glucose if used with secretagogues
Fenugreek	Diarrhea, gas; Uterine contractions; Allergic reactions	May increase anticoagulant effects of warfarin or herbs with anticoagulant activity (boldo, garlic, ginger)
Ginseng	Insomnia, headache, restlessness; Increase blood pressure or heart rate; Mastalgia; Mood changes, nervousness	Decrease warfarin effectiveness; Decrease diuretic effectiveness; Additive estrogenic effects; Possible increase effects of certain analgesics and antidepressants; Possible additive hypoglycemia with secretagogues
Gymnema	None reported; May cause hypoglycemia	Possible hypoglycemia if combined with secretagogues
	Diarrhea, weakness,	No adverse interactions known;

Milk Thistle	sweating; Possible allergic reactions if also allergic to ragweed, marigolds, daisies, chrysanthemums	Beneficial interactions with hepatotoxic agents such as acetaminophen, antipsychotics, alcohol
Nicotinamide	Headache; Skin reaction, allergies; GI upset; May trigger gout and peptic ulcer disease; May adversely affect liver function – monitor LFTs and platelet function	May increase serum concentrations of certain anticonvulsants
Nopal	Diarrhea, nausea, abdominal fullness; Increase stool volume	Improved blood glucose and insulin with sulfonylureas (without hypoglycemia)
Vanadium	GI upset; Animal research shows potential for accumulation	May potentiate anticoagulant effects of antiplatelet agents; May potentiate therapeutic or toxic effects of digoxin

American Association of Diabetes Educators "The Art and Science of Diabetes Self-Management Education. A Desk Reference for Healthcare Professionals" 2006.

Chapter 9

HOSPITALIZATION
Step by Step Guidelines

Research regarding inpatient treatment for patients with type 1 diabetes and eating disorders (ED-DMT1) is limited; guidelines are based on clinical experience and consensus of experts. The criteria for admission and steps of inpatient treatments have been gathered from multiple hospitals in treating patients with diabetic complications along with the complications of eating disorders.

Criteria for Hospitalization

- Diabetic ketoacidosis

- Dehydration

- Electrolyte imbalance (potassium 3.0 or less, phosphorus 3.0 or less, magnesium 1.8 or less)

- Hypothermia, body temperature below 36.3

- Orthostasis, on standing, pulse increase of more than 35bpm, systolic blood pressure decrease of more than 10, diastolic blood pressure drop of more than 10

- Bradycardia, heart rate below 50 the day, 45 at night

- Prolonged QTC interval on a electrocardiogram (QTC >0.45)

- Severe malnutrition (<75% median body weight for age)

Steps for Inpatient Treatment

Step 1: Stabilize the patient; eliminate the crisis.

The critical care team along with endocrinologists and the eating disorder team work immediately to establish metabolic control and vital signs stability.

Step 2: Evaluate the patient further via multi-disciplinary team management:

a. Medical consequences

If the patient has long standing diabetes (at least 4 post pubertal years of diabetes), the endocrinology team may evaluate diabetes complications caused by insulin manipulation. These include: Retinopathy, nephropathy, neuropathy or cardiac and gastrointestinal involvement.

The eating disorder side of diabulimia has serious complications as well, such as nutritional deficiency, amenorrhea (absence of menstrual period) and pubertal delay. Also, there is the potential of low bone mineral density, leading to osteoporosis and increased fracture risk.

b. Mental health risks.

It is essential that mental health complications and risk assessment be evaluated as well. Remember Brenda's story? Her parents saw no need for psychotherapy. They were not comfortable with the concept of Brenda having a mental illness. Some parents and ults ignore the referral from their primary care provider for psycho-social consult, even though some teens wish they could talk to someone about their problem. Being hospitalized gives them that opportunity, and it is invaluable.

Fortunately, there are effective mental health assessment tools available. Clinicians recommend:

Rosenberg Self-Esteem Scale

Eating Disorders Examination Questionnaire

Patient Health Questionnaire

Eating Disorders Inventory of Traits and Changes

These questionnaires aid in the diagnosis of ED-DMT1 and any other psychiatric co-morbidity, which then helps clinicians determine the appropriate course of treatment. However, they can not take the place of comprehensive assessment by experienced mental health clinicians.

c. Nutrition assessment

Meeting with a registered dietitian to establish medical nutrition therapy is an essential part of the treatment, it may start on day one of hospitalization.

Step 3: Monitor and educate the patient.

- **Be realistic about blood glucose goals**

Individuals who have been omitting insulin regularly are accustomed to living in a moderate to severe hyperglycemic state as a base-line. For them, being in a normal blood glucose range may cause symptoms of hypoglycemia such as headache, fatigue, dizziness or shakiness. The team should discuss a realistic blood glucose goal for each patient.

For example, if a patient's average blood glucose has been over 350mg/dL (HbA1c >14%) for the past three months, the goal should be <300mg/dL for the first few days, then adjusted to <250mg/dL for the next few days, with <200mg/dL as the goal.

- **Establish a blood glucose monitoring schedule.**

Ideally, patients with type 1 diabetes should be checking their blood glucose upon arising, before every meal and snack, and once or twice in the evening as well as overnight. The reality is that those who are admitted to the hospital with ED-DMT1 have usually not been checking their blood glucose regularly, if at all, for quite some time.

If a patient agrees to check blood glucose in the morning, prior to eating a big meal and before going to bed, just three times a day, that schedule is no doubt far superior to what the patient was doing before being hospitalized.

Taking responsibility away: Initially, the nursing staff takes the responsibility of conducting frequent blood glucose monitoring. Once the blood glucose goal is established and stabilized, the patient may work with a diabetes educator or a nurse to become educated about the optimal time and frequency of checking blood glucose at home. Some negotiation may be needed to gradually increase testing to the ideal frequency.

Giving responsibility back to the patient: A patient may earn the "privilege" of checking their own blood glucose on a reasonable home schedule as long as she/he is closely supervised. The process of educating the patient about medical consequences should be ongoing.

The inpatient setting is a highly effective classroom in which individuals can learn how many times and when to check their own blood glucose in order to keep it under control.

> IF PATIENTS HAVEN'T TAKEN RESPONSIBILITY FOR MONITORING THEIR OWN BLOOD GLUCOSE, THEY WILL HAVE TO EARN THE "PRIVILEGE" BACK, UNDER SUPERVISION.

- **Insulin pumps and patients with diabulimia**

Insulin administration needs to be performed by staff personnel initially. Some institutions may change the patient to multiple daily injections (MDI). If the patient is using a pump, the medical staff need to observe or administer all boluses, and the insulin pump should be uploaded every several days, and when insulin is delivered, the infusion set and infusion site should be observed to be sure the infusion set has not been disconnected.

When the patient is discharged, it may still be necessary to observe or have others administer insulin doses with either multiple daily injections therapy or insulin pump therapy. Some believe these patients should not resume giving their own insulin until they demonstrate improved HbA1c after a few follow up visits to the out patient diabetes clinic.

Insulin pumps allow the health personnel to review insulin delivery through a pump upload, however there are many ways a patient may "fake out" this system, such as disconnecting the infusion set before giving a bolus. This is why it is sometimes worthwhile to be sure that a minimal basal dose of insulin is given each day through the subcutaneous injection of a long acting insulin.

- **Multiple Daily Subcutaneous Insulin Therapy**

A common regimen of multiple daily insulin injections consists of the use of a long-acting basal insulin (such as Glargine or Detemir) once a day, combined with injections of rapid-acting insulin (such as Lispro, Aspart or Glulisine) when eating carbohydrates. Additional injections, referred to as correction boluses, become necessary when the blood glucose value is higher than the target for each individual.

- **The insulin regimen is individualized**

Long-acting basal insulins have a duration of 20 to 24 hours. Fast-acting insulins peak at 0.5 to 1.5 hours after injection, and last for 3 to 6 hours. The endocrinology team establishes a plan for basal insulin, insulin to carbohydrate ratio, and correction boluses for each patient. This individualized plan is based on such factors as each individual's blood glucose value, age, diabetes duration, insulin sensitivity and target blood glucose.

Prior to admission, individuals who suffer from diabulimia (ED-DMT1) may not have been taking bolus insulin at all. Since they tend to skip taking insulin before eating, and seldom check blood glucose, they don't make corrections with bolus insulin when their blood glucose is high. Quite often, they only take basal insulin to prevent diabetic ketoacidosis.

Again, the shift of responsibility takes place through the inpatient treatment. Initially the nursing staff takes over the insulin administration; next, the patient works toward giving their own insulin observed by the staff; and finally, the patient assumes responsibility for their own insulin administration, if applicable.

Jessica, age 22:
"I started skipping insulin when I was 13. I only took the basal insulin just to stay out of the emergency room. "

"I was diagnosed with type 1 diabetes when I was 11 years old. By the time I was 13, I was skipping insulin. I just didn't take it at school, and at home I lied to my Mom and told her I already took it in my room before dinner. I never even checked my blood glucose unless she was standing over me.

When she went back to work full time I was 15, and nobody was around to check up on me. My Dad didn't feel comfortable talking to me about diabetes. I even stopped taking the basal insulin at night and no one noticed. But then I started having DKA and had to go to the emergency room twice. That was horrible enough--I sure didn't want to be hospitalized.

It didn't take me long to figure out that if I just took basal insulin at night, I could skip the other insulin and not get DKA. I know it's a wonder I didn't kill myself. And I am now trying to get some help."

ALL JESSICA TOOK WAS BASAL INSULIN SO SHE COULD AVOID DIABETIC KETOACIDOSIS. NOW SHE IS DESPERATE FOR HELP.

Recap:

Nursing staff takes responsibility

Soon after metabolic and vital signs are stabilized, the nursing staff assumes all care including monitoring of blood glucose, and measuring and administration of insulin.

Patient/staff share responsibility

When the team agrees the patient is ready to take some responsibility, the nursing staff begins supervising and observing the patient's self-management.

Patient takes responsibility

Prior to discharge, the patient should be educated, and should have assumed some of, if not all responsibility for their own insulin administration and blood glucose monitoring. The need for supervision on discharge needs to be individualized.

- **Detecting and Minimizing Self-Induced Vomiting**

The fear of weight gain drives most patients with diabulimia to withhold insulin, but in the hospital, omitting insulin is not an option. Once manipulation of insulin is no longer possible, patients look for another compensatory behavior to lose weight, such as purging (self-induced vomiting).

Suspect purging when:

... laboratory results show high urine pH, high serum amylase or low serum potassium and/or high serum bicarbonate.

... patient's behavior includes going to the bathroom after eating, leaving faucet running.

... noises and smells may be present in the bathroom.

To minimize the purging behavior, the nursing staff may establish a one-to- one observation protocol one to two hours after meals or snacks.

- **Educating the patient.**

A diabetes education plan should include "survival skills education;" i.e. self treatment of symptoms such as hypoglycemia or hyperglycemia and self management of sick days.

Diabetes self-management education can be challenging during hospitalization. However, patients with diabulimia are known for not following up on self-management techniques once they go home. Diabetes educators, nursing staff and registered dietitians should take advantage of the situation while patients are in the hospital, providing and reviewing as much pertinent information as possible. This could be the patient's only opportunity to receive diabetes education.

A diabetes education should address weight management.

If patients are overweight, a registered dietitian should address effective weight control methods including choosing adequate portions, making healthy food choices, cooking at home, eating low calorie snacks and exercising.

> ▪ **What to do about weight gain.**
>
> It is almost inevitable that patients with diabetes will gain weight after receiving appropriate insulin administration, mostly because they are no longer losing glucose (and therefore calories) through the urine (glucosuria); i.e., the food is used in the cells instead of being lost in the urine.
>
> Initially, it may be better if the patient does not see the numbers on the scale. If patients insist, it's a good idea to weigh them prior to a psychotherapy session.
>
> However, at least a few days prior to discharge, it may be beneficial for patients to confront their weight and be able to work through their reactions with a team of professionals. This can minimize their reaction to seeing the numbers at home, which can trigger a relapse soon after being discharged.

Step 4: Make the transition to outpatient treatment

Patients should have follow-up appointments prior to discharge. Most diabetes clinics at major medical centers have multi-disciplinary team members. All appointments can be made at one center where the team members are capable of treating individuals with ED-DMT1, diabulimia.

Unfortunately, a high percentage of patients fail to follow through with their appointments. Chapter 10, entitled "What Works," will address ways to keep recovery going forward.

Chapter 10

WHAT WORKS, WHAT DOESN'T

How Individuals with Diabulimia Cheat

Those with diabulimia can be very clever. They secretly find ways to outsmart the system, their health care providers and their families in order to maintain control over their weight. It is crucial for families and health personnel to be able to detect these behaviors, and confront the individuals with the truth. That is the hope: If the behavior is recognized, and brought out into the open, it can be stopped before permanent damage is done. Look for:

- Counterfeiting glucose readings by substituting other liquids for blood on the test strip.

Patricia, age 16
"I convinced my mother my blood glucose readings were fine when they weren't."

"My mother was always asking to see the test strips for my blood glucose readings. What she didn't know was that I was using diluted juice instead of blood on the test strips so I would have a reading below the 200's. Then she started getting suspicious because my numbers were almost perfect most of the time. So I started to vary them sometimes by adding more juice to increase the number of the reading. I thought I was very clever, but the clinic figured it out."

THERE ARE WAYS TO FALSIFY THE BLOOD
GLUCOSE READING.

There are many other ways to counterfeit test results. The simplest way is to only test on "good days" when one thinks there will be a good result. Some people have used a "control" test solution on their meter strips, and others have used certain shades of nail polish. Also, some apply a smaller sample to get a lower reading, or dilute their blood before applying it to the strip. Another strategy is to have some residual alcohol on the finger when testing, because alcohol will inactivate the glucose oxidase enzyme in the strip and give a lower reading. Different ingenious ways to "falsify" test results work with different meters. As new meters are available, new ways to falsify results will be found.

- **Throwing away vials of insulin**

Often, families take the responsibility of getting insulin prescriptions filled whenever the supply of vials is running low. They may suspect something when insulin vials are not being used. Therefore some individuals throw away full vials to create the false impression that they are using the right amount of insulin. Of course those who live alone don't have to throw away the vials; they just leave them in the refrigerator unused.

Susan's Mom
"When I visited my daughter in her dorm room, the insulin vials were piled up in the fridge"

Susan's mother could plainly see how much her 22 year old daughter was struggling. On one visit to her college dorm, she found Susan curled up in a ball in the corner of her room. It broke her heart to see how tired and nauseous her daughter had become. In the refrigerator, there seemed to be the same amount of insulin as there had been two weeks ago. Obviously Susan wasn't taking her insulin and was suffering all the symptoms of hyperglycemia.

- **Forgetting to bring meters to the doctor's office**

Those who aren't taking enough insulin try to conceal it. They don't want the doctor to know they haven't been checking their blood glucose often enough, or how high their readings have been. The meter reveals not only blood glucose levels, but also the times and dates when the levels were checked. So when it's time to see the doctor, these individuals conveniently "forget" to bring the meter, or claim the meter has been lost or broken.

- **"Injecting" insulin outside the skin when under observation**

What about individuals who are under strict observation in the hospital, at school or at home in order to get their blood glucose under control? Unless they are carefully watched, they may only pretend to inject insulin, while in reality letting it drip outside the skin. Some individuals have been known to inject the insulin into a couch or mattress while the parent looks away. The family member or health personnel will not be able to detect this unless standing within an arm's length of the individual.

Another method of giving an inadequate dose of insulin is to withdraw air from the insulin bottle instead of insulin. In the syringe air and insulin look the same since Lantus and analog short acting insulin are clear. So even if care takers or nurses are checking the syringe for the correct dosage, they will not know that air is been given.

- **Cheating when using an insulin pump**

An insulin pump is programmed to deliver a small amount of basal insulin every few minutes through a tube that is connected to an insulin reservoir inside the pump. But in addition to having the basal insulin, the users need to initiate bolus doses of insulin before meals or to correct high blood glucose levels.

Most individuals with diabulimia intentionally do not "tell" the pump to deliver the bolus doses. In some severe cases, they even unplug the connection between the insulin reservoir and the skin and let the basal insulin drip outside of the skin. That way a bolus delivery is recorded on the pump.

Some do not use the meter that links with their pump and instead, enter false blood sugar numbers manually in their pump, so it appears like they are testing. Some consistently manipulate the dates in the meter so when the meter is downloaded the dates do not correlate with the pump information.

Regardless of how they modify meter and insulin logs or pump downloads; the HbA1c will reflect the true average blood glucose over the previous two to three months. That is one reason why many of those who manipulate insulin are reluctant to see doctors. They do not want to be confronted with their true blood glucose values.

> THOSE WHO HAVE BEEN CHEATING WITH METERS OR AN INSULIN PUMP DO NOT WANT TO BE CONFRONTED WITH THEIR TRUE BLOOD GLUCOSE VALUES, SO THEY TRY TO AVOID DOCTORS.

Why are those with diabulimia so determined to hide the fact that they are not taking their insulin? Why do they go to such lengths to trick clinicians and their families? They conceal their sad secret as long as they possibly can. When *Carolyn* was confronted with her behavior she became angry and resistant, shouting *"This is the only weapon I have left to fight gaining weight! You can't take it away from me!"*

What can families and health personnel do to help those who suffer with diabulimia? Does anything work? Yes, but first, let's look at what doesn't work:

What doesn't work?

- **Scare tactics do not work.**

One provider said to Kali, age 20

> *"Unless you start taking care of yourself, you will be on dialysis by the time you're 30! You'll have nerve damage and your feet will have to be chopped off!"*

Kali's response?

"Don't worry; I'll kill myself by then."

- **Guilt trips do not work.**

One frustrated father told his daughter, Michaela, age 14

> *"Look, if you don't shape up, you'll wind up in the hospital again. Is that what you want? Your mother and I spent a lot of money getting tickets to Disney World. Your brother has never even been there! Don't ruin our vacation just because you don't want to take insulin!"*

Michaela's reply:

"Just go ahead without me. I don't care. I would rather be home by myself or in a hospital than on vacation with you anyway."

- **"Put-downs" and belittling do not work**

A mother said to her daughter Stephanie, age 17

"How can an A student be so stupid! Don't you have any common sense? Don't you even know what you are doing to your body?"

Stephanie replied:

"It's my body, and I can do whatever I want with it!"

WHAT DOESN'T WORK:

SCARE TACTICS

GUILT TRIPS

PUT-DOWNS

> EVERYBODY HAS SOMETHING OF VITAL
> IMPORTANCE TO THEM.

WHAT WORKS?

I. Learn What Motivates Those with Diabulimia: Find the Hot Button

What is it that is vitally important?

Success in helping individuals make progress depends on learning what motivates them. There is always something vitally important to everyone; it's up to clinicians and families to find out what it is. One might think that preventing limb amputation, blindness, renal dialysis, or death would be highly motivational. However, most teenagers and young adults don't seem to think any of that could happen to them; it's just too far away. They are far more likely to be motivated by immediate gratification and social consequences.

Pre-teens want to grow taller

A study in 2006 indicated that in children with type 1 diabetes, height is strongly correlated with proper glycemic control. If someone has not yet attained full growth, any manipulation of insulin that worsens the glucose control can stunt growth and reduce potential height. Pre-teens do not want to be short!

Admonishing a 11 year old to "make sure you take your insulin or you'll damage your health" may not sink in. However, informing her that without enough insulin she could be stunting her growth may set off an alarm. Say "You'll keep growing if you keep your blood glucose in a good range by taking your insulin." Once she knows she can't reach her full height unless her body gets the insulin it needs, she may be motivated to take it.

Older teens want to go to a good college

Fatigue, tiredness and headaches are common symptoms of hyperglycemia. These do not lead to clear thinking. A good student will try anything to have more energy and a longer attention span in order to get better grades and be accepted at a good college.

Talk to students about keeping their blood glucose under control with proper insulin to prevent fatigue and increase energy. This will be more motivational than telling them about the complications of diabetes.

Athletes wish to build muscle mass

Once an athlete learns that insulin helps to promote protein synthesis and preserve lean body mass, he or she may become very motivated to take adequate insulin for better performance.

Young adults wish to be healthy to have babies

High hemoglobin A1c levels and being underweight may cause irregular menses or amenorrhea (cessation of menses). Not having menses or ovulation can be an important issue to someone who is becoming interested in dating, marriage and having a family. Wanting to have a baby can be a huge driving force to motivate good self-care and better controlled blood glucose.

Cindy, age 25
"I feel like a 55 year old woman, I need to get help and get my periods back"
"I have done so much damage to my body because of diabulimia that I feel more like 55 years old instead of 25 years old. I had missed my periods since I was 18. I am now married; my husband and I desperately wish to have our own children. "

Parents want to take good care of their children

Most parents feel responsible for their children's well being. They are willing to make sacrifices and do whatever it takes to care for them. They may not be concerned about taking good care of themselves, but they are concerned about feeling well enough to take good care of their children. Once they understand that without proper blood glucose control they cannot be healthy parents, they may be motivated to take the right amount of insulin.

Hard workers hate to miss work

Those with a good work ethic and a desire to succeed do not want to be incapacitated. Symptoms of hyperglycemia such as nausea or severe headaches can make them miss valuable work time. A great motivator for hard workers is to understand that a proper insulin regime keeps them feeling well, which helps them in the work place.

People choose to be free from physical pain

When it comes to the quality of life, freedom from physical pain is more important than a high income, according to a 2010 survey in a metropolitan area. Peripheral neuropathy due to diabetic complications can lead to excruciating pain. Those who have ever had to experience it would gladly take adequate insulin to make the pain go away, if it's not too late. Preventing painful neuropathy has to be proactive, by choosing to take insulin and keeping HbA1c below 7%.

Most people can't stand the thought of losing their eyesight

Having clear eyesight is a powerful motivator. When blood glucose stays over 250mg/dL for a week, the lenses of the eyes swell due to osmotic change. This causes blurred vision, which, fortunately, is reversible. However, the eyesight could be permanently damaged if the hyperglycemia is prolonged.

The possibility of going blind is more frightening to some people than losing a kidney. Talking about how to protect vision and prevent loss of eyesight may be a highly effective approach.

EVERYBODY HAS A HOT BUTTON:

FULL GROWTH. GOOD GRADES .
ATHLETICISM. FERTILITY .
FREEDOM FROM PAIN.
CONCERN FOR CHILDREN.
CAREER. EYESIGHT.

IT'S UP TO CLINICIANS AND FAMILIES
TO FIND THAT VITAL MOTIVATOR .

---

2. Setting Small Goals Works.

It's overwhelming for those who have diabulimia when health care providers or caretakers expect them to accept the full amount of insulin prescribed. The less insulin they had been taking, the higher their HbA1c became, and the more insulin was prescribed at the next visit. Therefore, the gap between what was prescribed and what was taken actually widened.

Observe them taking basal insulin

Those who have been treated as outpatients may not have taken insulin at all. For better compliance, meet them where they are. Start at small doses and increase slowly. The first step is to start with basal insulin. If they are on multiple daily injections (MDI) therapy, then have them take the basal insulin once a day at first, while being observed by a family member.

If the individual is using an insulin infusion pump, upload the insulin pump and review their basal and bolus doses. Work with them to decide on a reasonable carbohydrate to insulin ratio, review times of missed meal boluses, and consider increasing basal insulin if there are consistent periods of hyperglycemia during the day.

When there are frequent pump suspensions or temporary decreases in the basal rate, consider adding a dose of long acting insulin equivalent to the patient's minimal basal rate multiplied by 24. Next, subtract this minimal hourly basal rate from each hour to create a new basal rate pattern. The caretaker can then administer the basal insulin, or carefully observe the individual self-administer this basal insulin each day. Although this measure will prevent one from going into ketoacidosis, in itself, it cannot accomplish overall good diabetes control, which can only be achieved by the appropriate delivery of insulin at meals.

Check blood glucose and make corrections

Those with diabulimia need to be empowered by making decisions. Let them choose the time they wish to check their blood glucose, but without negotiating the frequency. For example: be firm in requiring that they check blood glucose twice a day, but have them choose what time they want to do the checking. Slowly work up to three times a day, and ideally at least four times a day.

To go from checking twice a day to four times a day is a gradual process that may take a few weeks or even a few months. This is because every time individuals with diabulimia check their blood glucose and find their level is higher than the target range, they will be expected to take a correction dose of insulin. This behavior can be verified when individuals use an insulin pump download. However, there is currently no way to know whether or not the individuals are taking correction doses of insulin if they are using syringes or insulin pens.

Bolus Insulin for Carbohydrate Intakes

Working on bolus insulin doses is the last step in the outpatient treatment of diabulimia. Some take several months to get to this step because they don't want to face how much they eat and how much insulin they need to take for carbohydrates.

The goal is to decrease blood glucose slowly over time. Some clinicians believe that decreasing by 10mg/dL per week is a good goal (outside the hospital).

Kelly's story, age 16
"I was afraid to gain weight. I was afraid to take insulin. I was just afraid. "

Kelly was terrified of weight gain. When she first came to the clinic, she wasn't even taking insulin. She had been prescribed 30U of basal insulin at night plus insulin to carbohydrate ratio of 1:15. She was overwhelmed so she took nothing. There was no way she would go from nothing to full compliance, so she was asked to start out with 5U of basal insulin at night. She agreed to do that much. Then we asked her to increase it 5U every week and she complied. It wasn't until a month later that she agreed to check her blood glucose twice a day and make corrections. Three months later, she finally agreed to begin adding insulin for her carbohydrate intake. Very slow progress, but progress in the right direction.

3. Helping to Develop a Healthy Life Style Works

Establish sound eating habits

Helping individuals to develop healthy eating behavior is the foundation for recovery from diabulimia. Helping those who are overweight to obtain steady weight loss by improving their lifestyle is paramount. Highlights of sound eating habits include having proper portions; incorporating high quality nutrients, and making low calorie food choices; having a good breakfast and healthy snacks; planning a realistic meal schedule; and developing simple recipes for homemade meals.

Prevent binge eating

The cycle of food deprivation followed by binging is vicious. Drastically restricting food causes symptoms of hypoglycemia, which causes hunger, which leads to overeating, which leads to manipulation of insulin. A sound meal schedule can eliminate the cycle. Skipping meals is the culprit that leads to grazing throughout the day, and mindlessly racking up far more calories than three healthy meals would contain. Some eat "low carb" foods randomly, not taking into consideration that a few slices of cheese, or spoonfuls of peanut butter on celery and some handfuls of nuts add up to a significant amount of calories. Having three balanced meals and choosing snacks wisely is the basic principle in the prevention of binge eating.

Shift focus away from weight

Weight issues are at the core of eating disorders, and are covered throughout this book. Please refer to weight measurement: the pros and cons of revealing body weight to those with diabulimia, in Chapter 7. In general, it's better to focus on healthy lifestyle and not body weight.

Promote appropriate exercise

With the exception of those who are underweight, who have unstable vital signs, or who exhibit compulsive exercise behavior, appropriate physical activities can be usefully integrated into the diabulimia treatment plan. With hypoglycemia precaution in place, thirty to forty minutes of low to moderate impact exercise four to five times a week is optimal.

4. Continuing Education Works

In the world of cyberspace, individuals are bombarded with information. They may be negatively influenced by internet chat rooms or blogs. They may browse through various websites and only pick up on the statements they want to believe.

For health personnel, persistence is the key to educating this population. It's like moving a mountain, one shovel full at a time. Giving up is not an option. At each meeting, educate on one subject. Simply provide education without judgment, without a sales pitch, and without scare tactics. Sooner or later, the mountain of misinformation will become diminished while a structure of sound education grows tall and strong.

Listen to the voice of diabulimia.

People with diabulimia may feel different. They live in a world where nobody else has to poke their finger a few times a day. Nobody else has to worry about taking insulin when they eat. Some with diabulimia believe they can never be "normal"; some grieve for the days when they "were healthy."

They hear people lecturing them, criticizing them, telling them what to do, thwarting the only way they know to avoid their fear: weight gain. They think nobody knows what it's like to have diabetes and "to be fat". What they need is understanding.

The best thing families and health personnel can give them is a sympathetic ear. Take the time to listen. Listen to their fear, their struggle; and especially, listen to their cry for help.

An Outcry for Self and for Others

Lucy, age 40

"I am forty and have been battling an eating disorder and diabetes for twenty-five years. I skip shots and have numerous diabetes complications. I now use a wheelchair because of a foot ulcer and neuropathy. I have no hope now, but those younger people do. Please help them somehow! When I tried to find help, I didn't know where to turn. There were no resources--I could not find a single book that addressed this terrible thing. Please do something to help the young ones so they will never have to live like this. "

REFERENCES

Achard DM, Vik N, Neumark-Sztainer D. et al. Disordered eating and body dissatisfaction in adolescents with type 1 diabetes and a population-based comparison sample: comparative prevalence and clinical implications. Pediatr Diabetes. 2008;28(4 pt 1):312-9.

American Diabetes Association: "Standard of Medical Care in Diabetes – 2010" Diabetes Care. 2010;33:S11-61.

American Diabetes Association and American Dietetic Association: Choose Your Foods: Exchange Lists for Diabetes.

American Association of Diabetes Educators "The Art and Science of Diabetes Self-Management Education. A Desk Reference for Healthcare Professionals" 2006.

American Psychiatric Association: Diagnostic and Statistical Manual of Mental Disorders. 4th Ed. Washington, D.C., American Psychiatric Association, 2000

Antisdel JE. Improved detection of eating problems in women with type1 diabetes using a newly developed survey. Diabetes. 2001;50(S1):A47.

Bantle JP, Wylie-Rosett J, Albright AL, et al. Nutrition recommendations and interventions for diabetes: a position statement of the American Diabetes Association. Diabetes Care 2008;31(S1):S61-78.

Bermudez O, Gallivan H, Jahraus J, et al. Inpatient management of eating disorders in type 1 diabetes. Diabetes Spectrum. 2009;22(3):153-158.

Bryden KS, Neil A, Mayou, RA, et al. Eating habits, body weight, and insulin misuse. A longitudinal study of teenagers and young adults with type 1 diabetes. Diabetes Care. 1999; 22:1956-1960.

Cantwell R, Steel, JM. Screening for eating disorders in diabetes mellitus. J of Psychosomatic Research. 1996;40(1)15-20.

Chase PC, Messer L. Understanding insulin pumps & continuous glucose monitors. 2nd edition 2010. Children's Diabetes Foundation at Denver, Colorado.

Colton PA, Olmsted MP, Daneman, D, et al. Natural history and predictors of disturbed eating behavior in girls with type 1 diabetes. Diabet Med 2007; 24:424-9.

Colton P, Rodin G, Bergenstal R, et al. Eating disorders and diabetes: introduction and overview. 2009;22(3):138-142.

Crigeo A, Crow S, Goebel-Fabbri A, et al. Eating disorders and diabetes: screening and detection. Diabetes Spectrum. 2009;22(3):143-146.

Dahan A, McAfee SG. A proposed role for the psychiatrist in the treatment of adolescents with type 1 diabetes mellitus. Psychiatr Q.2009;80(2):75-85.

DAFNE Study Group. Training in flexible, intensive insulin management to enable dietary freedom in people with type 1 diabetes: dose adjustment for normal eating (DAFNE) randomized controlled trial. BMJ. 2002;325:746-52.

Daneman D, Olmsted M, Rydall, A, et al. Eating disorders in young women with type 1 diabetes : prevalence, problems and prevention. Hormone Research. 1998;50:79-86.

Elamin A, Hussin O, Tuvemo T. Growth, puberty and final height in children with type 1 diabetes. J Diabetes Complications. 2006;20(4):252-6.

Evert A, Gerken S. Birth through adolescences. In diabetes medical nutrition therapy and education. American Dietetic Association. 2005:161-78.

Fairburn CG, Steel JM. Anorexia nervosa in diabetes mellitus. BMJ. 1980;280:1167-1168. (early report in 1980's)

Goebel-Fabbri A. Disturbed eating behaviors and eating disorders in type 1 diabetes; clinical significance and treatment recommendations. Current Diabetes Report. 2009;9:133-139.

Goebel-Fabbri A, Fikkan J, Connell A, et al. Identification and treatment of eating disorders in women with type 1 diabetes mellitus. Treat Endocrinol. 2002;1(3):155-162.

Goebel-Fabri A, Fikkan J, Franko D, et al. Insulin restriction and associated morbidity and mortality in women with type1 diabetes. Diabetes Care. 2008;31(3):415-9.

Goebel-Fabbri AE, Uplinger N, Gerken S, et al. Outpatient management of eating disorders in type 1 diabetes. Diabetes Spectrum. 2009;22(3):147-152.

Gomez J, Dally P, Isaacs AJ. Anorexia nervosa in diabetes mellitus. BMU. **1980**;281:61-62.

Hasken J, Kresl L, Nydegger T, et al. Diabulimia and the role of school health personnel. J Sch Health. 2010;80(10):465-9.

Hillard JR, Lobo MC, Keeling RP. Bulimia and diabetes: a potentially life-threatening combination. Psychosomatics. 1983.:24:292-295. **(provided comprehensive description of the complications of eating disorders and type 1 diabetes in early 1980's).**

Hoffman RP. Eating disorders in adolescents with type 1 diabetes, a closer look at a complicated condition. Postgrad Med. 2001;109(4):67-9, 73-4.

Influence of intensive diabetes treatment on body weight and composition and adults with type 1 diabetes in the Diabetes Control and Complications Trail. Diabetes Care 2001;24:1911-21.

Institute of Medicine: Dietary Reference Intakes: Energy, Carbohydrate, Fiber, Fat, Fatty Acids, Cholesterol, Protein, Vitamins and Elements. Washington, DC: National Academics Press; 2010.

Jaser SS. Psychological problems in adolescents with diabetes. Adolesc Med State Art Rev. 2010;21(1);138-51.

Kakleas K, Kandyla B, Karayianni C, et al. Psychosocial problems in adolescents with type 1 diabetes mellitus. Diabetes Metab. 2009;35(5):339-50.

Krause's Food, Nutrition & Diet Therapy, 12th edition. 2009. WB Saunders Company.

Lacey K, Pritchett E. Nutrition care process and model: ADA adopts road map to quality care and outcomes management. J Am Diet Assoc. 2003;103:1061-72.

Lustman PJ, Anderson RJ, Freedland KE, et al. Depression and poor glycemic control: a meta-analytic review of the literature. Diabetes Care 2000; 23:934-42.

Markowitz JT, Butler DA, Volkening LK, et al. Brief screening tool for disordered eating in diabetes: internal consistency and external validity in a contemporary sample of pediatric patients with type 1 diabetes. Diabetes Care. 2010;33(3):495-500.

Markowitz JT, Lowe MR, Volkening LK, et al. Self reported history of overweight and its relationship to disordered eating in adolescent girls with type 1 diabetes. Diabet Med. 2009;26(11):1165-71.

McMurry, JE: Organic Chemistry, 8th edition. 2008. Thomas Brooks/Cole Pub Co.

Mehta SN, Quinn N, Volkening LK, et al. Impact of carbohydrate counting on glycemic control in children with type 1 diabetes. 2009;32(6):1014-1016.

Melendez-Ramirez LY, Richards RJ, Cefalu WT. Complications of type 1 diabetes. Endocrinol Metab Clin North Am. 2010;39(3):625-40.

Author: **Grace Huifeng Shih, RD, MS**
Registered dietitian with diabetes team, Lucile Packard Children's Hospital
(**LPCH**), Stanford Medical Center; Board member of Eating Disorder Resource
Center (**EDRC**); Speaker for eating disorders and diabulimia workshops; Private
practice nutritionist who educates clients with diabulimia in her four offices
throughout Northern California

Editor: **Bruce Buckingham, MD**
Endocrinologist at LPCH and Professor at Stanford University, Palo Alto, CA

Editor: **Rosanna Fiallo-Scharer, MD**
Endocrinologist at Barbara Davis Center and Associate Professor at
University of Colorado, Denver, CO
****

"This book is a must read for individuals struggling with diabulimia, a highly
complex and misunderstood condition which causes sufferers to feel isolated
and alone. The author does a beautiful job of blending insightful anecdotes with
solid research and expertise to keep the reader engaged throughout the book. I
highly recommend it."
Tonja H. Krautter, Psy.D., LCSW
Author of *What Every Parent Needs to Know about Eating Disorders*; Radio and
TV spokesperson who discusses difficult matters such as eating disorders

"Grace Shih's elaborate writing about diabulimia is so comprehensive and
informative. I want to make this superb book a must-read resource for the loved
ones of those who suffer from diabulimia and for professionals who interact with
this dual diagnosis."
Seham El-Diwany, MD
Pediatrician; Board member of Eating Disorders Coalition and EDRC

"Using a series of vivid patient vignettes, Grace Shih illuminates when to suspect
diabulimia, an often hidden clinical problem. In this book, she outlines many of
the signs of symptoms that are associated with this eating disorder as well as
approaches to modifying this behavior. Health personnel, families and
Individuals will find this book a very helpful guide to such a challenging
condition."
Darrell Wilson, MD
Director, Pediatrics Division of Endocrinology & Diabetes, LPCH; Professor,
Stanford University.

Made in the USA
San Bernardino, CA
18 November 2014